The Shocking Reality of America's Healthcare

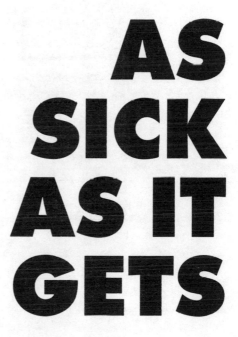

AS SICK AS IT GETS

A Diagnosis and Treatment Plan by

Rudolph Mueller M.D.

31

The Shocking Reality of
America's Healthcare

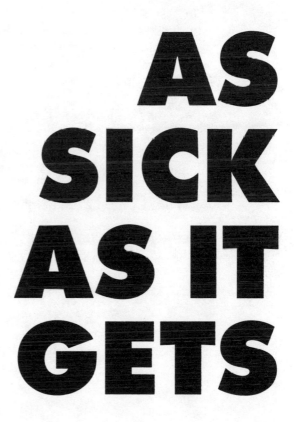

AS
SICK
AS IT
GETS

A Diagnosis and
Treatment Plan by

Rudolph Mueller M.D.

Olin Frederick, Inc.
Dunkirk, New York

Library of Congress Cataloging-in Publication Data
Mueller, Rudolph

As Sick as it Gets / Rudolph Mueller

ISBN: 0-9672357-8-2

362.1
muE

Printed in Canada

For Diane, my wife,
and Daniel, Nicholas, Theodore, Peter,
and Heidi,
with heartfelt thanks for all their love,
patience and support in this effort.

In memory of:

Dr. Richard P. Mueller
Dr. Walter P. Bass
Cadet David Bass, USAF

I also greatly appreciate so many people who have helped me along in this journey, namely, Diane, Cynthia, Sam, Rolly, Tom, Karen, Holly, Pat, Andy, Flo, Shirley, Glenn, Dick, Rosemary, Don, Sandy, Sharon, Marilyn, Tad, Nancy, Richard, Rusty, Luz, Cherish, Brian, Ross, Joan, Betty, Quint, Margaret, Jim, and Gerry.

CONTENTS

INTRODUCTION

"Of all of the forms of Inequality, injustice in healthcare is the most shocking and inhumane."

The Reverend Martin Luther King, Jr.

This is the story of the American healthcare system at the turn of the millennium from my perspective as a primary care and geriatric physician. There are stark realities about healthcare in America. This book is about the realities. It reveals that millions of Americans are sick because they are denied primary and preventive healthcare. It speaks of the pharmaceutical companies, and the more constructive role they could play. It describes the insurance industry and health maintenance organizations (HMOs) interfering on a daily basis with patient care and harassing doctors and hospitals with wasteful administrative requirements. It tells of greed permeating the system and the confusing and demoralizing effects it has on the caregivers and their associates. It compares the American system to the next nine largest industrialized democratic nations and shows Americans pay 58% more per capita for healthcare and suffer worse health than the average citizen of these nations. It gives the human and economic justification for a landmark change in public policy. At the end it calls for a national healthcare program that will rein in rampaging costs, reinstate quality, rebuild confidence and respect, and restore social justice.

There is ill will and controversy among America's healthcare professionals. In nursing, fewer students are entering the field while experienced nurses retire prematurely or leave patient care altogether.[1] Surveys show that a third or more of senior physicians plan early retirement or a change in career in the next three years.[2] Many other practitioners consider the American system to be sick and in need of major reform and restructuring. A recent CBS News poll has reported the American people feel the same way.[3] Many caregivers are disgusted with the greed, waste, and excesses they see daily. For individual Americans, healthcare costs continue to rise, creating economic hardship and concerns over access to proper care for themselves and their families. Corporations and businesses feel the same cost increases and continually face decisions regarding insurance benefits for their employees.

Except for the United States, all democratic, industrialized nations of the Organization for Economic Cooperation and Development (OECD), and in some developing nations, healthcare is considered a human right.[4] Those societies validate that right by providing all people with access to healthcare. This is woefully not true in the United States. In this country medical care is not a right; rather it is a service based on market-driven principles.

The healthcare industry and its lobbying organizations and many caregivers fiercely maintain that the American delivery system is the very best in the world because it is based on market-driven principles. They continually criticize other nations' health programs, which are essentially publicly financed and government guaranteed. They want Americans to believe that any change in their health system that includes more government involvement would court disaster, deprive Americans of quality medical care and constrain choice. They allege that government involvement will interfere with research and technology advances. This perception has been established by what is possibly the most extensive and costly combination in American history of a long-term public affairs program and government lobbies at the national and state levels. Elements of the industry oppose any universal program that would provide quality, affordable, accessible healthcare for all Americans. Through its influence, long cultivated in state legislatures and in Washington, the healthcare industry has garnered political control of issues relating to it.

The apparent motives are singularly related to the mammoth cash flow that streams toward the insurance companies, HMOs, pharmaceutical companies, and for-profit hospitals and providers. Healthcare is now the largest industry in every developed nation. In the United States, revenues reached $1,077.1 billion in 1998, the last year for which comprehensive data are available.[5] In 1998 Americans paid $4,178 per capita for healthcare or nearly 40% more than the next most expensive country, Switzerland, where it was $2,794 per capita. The American total expenditure on healthcare was 13.6% of Gross Domestic Product (GDP) in 1998. The next nine largest industrialized democracies spent a weighted average of 8.43% of their GDP. The excess paid by Americans was $428 billion, 43% more than the U.S. defense budget.[6] This raises a huge question: Where does this excess money go? Americans are not healthier than the Germans, Canadians or French. They are notably less healthy. In terms of total results, the U.S. health system ranks 37th in the

world, as measured by the World Health Organization, the worst performance of any affluent democratic nation.[7]

This mediocre performance and high cost raise another question: Does
a profit-motivated or market-driven system deliver high quality care for every
American or does it deliver high profits for those in the industry who seek
profit? The market-driven concept, in fact, brings inherent injustices to the
people of the United States, allowing 43 million Americans to live without
health insurance.[8] Nearly the same number of people are underinsured creating a healthcare "underclass" in this nation. This underclass comprises real
people with feelings, hopes, dreams, joys and sorrows. These individuals
must struggle to maintain their health or cope with illness without adequate
resources to do so.[9] Nearly 11 million children are being raised without
health insurance, and many will fail to obtain even basic health needs.[10]
Uninsured children and adults pass in and out of the system, and in the end,
some of them become needlessly sick.

When people of any age lack access to preventive or even basic healthcare, diseases can progress unabated, leading to more costly emergency
hospitalizations, and to premature disability and death. In the case of diabetes, cardiovascular diseases and cancer, early treatment prevents disability
and saves lives. Prevention can be dramatically less expensive than later-
stage interventions. This system failure also inflicts large indirect costs on
families and society. The only way to save money by not providing basic
healthcare to all people in this nation is to not treat the consequent diseases
and let patients in the underclass die quickly and quietly outside the hospital and the system. In the United States over 200,000 people die annually
without seeing a doctor during the previous year.[11]

Others in the underclass, however, do not die quietly of preventable illnesses. They become desperate and seek care for themselves and their families
from hospitals, clinics, and doctors willing to treat them or who are required
to do so. If they become impoverished by their illnesses, they fall into the
welfare and Medicaid "safety net." If they survive to age sixty-five or are disabled, they qualify for Medicare and then are eligible to have much of their
high medical expenses paid.

The United States is carrying the burden of an unnecessary number of
sick people, a burden that could have been prevented with a universal health
system. This book will show that the cost of treatment for Americans who are
sick and who should not be sick represents a significant portion of the cost
excess between the United States and other OECD nations. It is on the twin
pillars of human need and cost savings that I base my call for universal, quality, affordable healthcare for the people in America with the freedom to
choose their own doctor, hospital, or other provider. It will prove to be a

monumental controversy.

The premise of this book is that the American healthcare system is sick, As Sick As It Gets. It is a system with a confused purpose and mission, contaminated by its focus on money and its exploitation of the massive cash flow that modern medical technology has created. Its mission should be to maximize the well-being and health of every individual and our society as a whole, as well as to prevent illness and to relieve pain. Every government in the OECD, except the American, has taken steps to grant the right of healthcare to every citizen, and in the process, preempt exploitation of healthcare and sick people.

This book includes the true stories of real-life illnesses of people who cannot afford adequate healthcare or who are denied it and my everyday experiences with them. It also includes stories about the system, the pharmaceutical industry, the insurance industry and HMOs, and the providers. These accounts are from one practice of one primary care physician over a two-year period in the United States. The names used in the stories are pseudonyms.

With the help of the staff of Olin-Frederick, I have done my best to give an accurate accounting of the human suffering and the related tragedy, and provide an analysis of where the excess money goes. I have made specific recommendations and outlined a detailed economic justification for a National Health Program that will heal the sickness of American healthcare.

Rudolph J. Mueller, MD
Jamestown, New York
October, 2001

1: THE UNINSURED

"Suppose a man comes into your meeting wearing a gold ring and fine clothes, and a poor man in shabby clothes also comes in. If you show special attention to the man wearing fine clothes and say, 'Here's a good seat for you,' but say to the poor man, 'You stand there' or 'Sit on the floor by my feet,' have you not discriminated among yourselves and become judges with evil thoughts?"
James 2: 2-4, The Holy Bible, The New International Version

By census estimates in 1999, the United States had nearly 43 million people who were living without health insurance.[1] Who are these uninsured millions? Over 75% of America's uninsured have full-time jobs or live in a household where at least one person is working full time.[2] One-fifth of the uninsured reside in homes where two or more employed adults live. Nearly one-third of the poor, one-third of Hispanics, and one-fifth of African-Americans are uninsured. Being uninsured is clearly related to household income, as 24% of households with incomes of less than $25,000 are uninsured compared to 8% of households with incomes over $75,000.[3]

These statistics are merely "numbers" and they utterly fail to show the complete reality. One high-level HMO official unemotionally stated to me, "There are only three million uninsured people in New York State." I tried to remind him these uninsured people are real human beings who suffer from unnecessary illness, premature disability, and early death. They are part of the healthcare "underclass" in the United States who lack timely access to preventive and primary levels of care and thereby suffer needless illness. Some are my patients, and I will share their stories throughout this book. Most of the 270,000 primary care physicians in this country have similar patients with similar stories, whether they realize it or not.

Over one hundred different medical studies document that uninsured patients suffer worse medical outcomes compared to the insured.[4] Nearly four of ten uninsured working-age adults failed to see any doctor in the previous year compared to less than one out of ten insured people. The chronically uninsured people in poor health fared even worse, with seven out of ten failing to see any doctor in the previous year.[5] As a practicing physician, I believe this is just plain bad medicine and exactly opposite of what any rational health system should provide. With our current system, patients in poor health see a doctor less often than those in good health.

When hospitalized, the uninsured are two to three times more likely to die than the insured because they seek and receive care later in the course of their illnesses, unlike "the more fortunate" insured patients.[6] The uninsured also undergo fewer cancer screening tests, including Pap smears, mammograms, or sigmoidoscopies, each shown to increase early detection and reduce cancer mortality rates.[7] But these are only medical studies and statistics of the uninsured. The poignant reality is revealed in their stories.

Terminal Cervical Cancer

I met Emily, a patient in the emergency room, when she presented critically ill. She was emaciated and yellow with jaundice. When I saw her I thought immediately of concentration camp victims. I found a large mass in her lower abdomen and suspected it was cancer. Further tests confirmed this, and showed the cancer was advanced and untreatable.

In the hospital I talked with Emily and told her what I had found. She then told me about how she had been uninsured for nearly ten years. She had left her employment to remain at home and care for her ailing father who later died. When I listened to her talk about him, it was obvious how much she loved her father. Unfortunately, Emily failed to see a doctor during her years of being uninsured, and sadly, now it was too late. A simple Pap smear a few years earlier could have saved her life.

"Why didn't you see a doctor sooner?" I asked her. Uninsured, Emily had two reasons why she delayed seeking care earlier—her fear of cancer and her fear of medical bills. She told me she would have seen a doctor sooner if she had insurance. She died only three days after admission to the hospital. Premature death is a common occurrence for the uninsured who present late in the course of their illness.

A Hypertensive Diabetic

Sam, a rugged working farmer, arrived in the emergency room by ambulance late one evening. The emergency room doctor consulted me for further management of this patient. Sam was self-employed, married and uninsured. He knew he had high blood pressure and possible "sugar" but had been treating it with herbs. He had not seen a doctor in nearly two years.

After working in the barn, Sam suddenly started coughing up pinkish phlegm and gasping for air. He thought it was merely a cold. Sam's vital signs were critically unstable. His skin was a dark blue in color from inadequate oxygen entering his bloodstream as a result of fluid-filled lungs. He nearly died from heart failure that night, but intravenous medications took hold and turned the precarious situation around. The untreated high blood pressure and diabetes, however, had already done considerable damage. Urgent cardiac testing at a larger medical center was required. I spent considerable time convincing Sam and his family of the necessity for additional tests and hospital treatments. I know they were concerned about the costs and possible need for cardiac surgery.

They mentioned herbal therapy and chelation treatments, all forms of Complementary and Alternative Medicine (CAM), for which many uninsured and insured patients turn to in times of need.[8] I was able to convince them that Sam was too critical and unstable for these forms of treatment. Thankfully, Sam survived this illness, but for how long? One shudders to think how many people are suffering the consequences of untreated chronic medical conditions.

Too many uninsured patients show up too late and too sick. Despite the growth of managed care, emergency room visits keep climbing. There are many reasons for this increase including lack of access to primary care doctors, especially among the poorest urban and rural communities, and uninsured patients. The Common Wealth Fund, a private philanthropic organization, found 75% of all emergency room visits in New York City were for non-emergencies. A spokesman for the American College of Emergency Physicians stated, "The situation is grave. We are a symptom of the disease that is the healthcare system."[9] In the United States, the only places where patients have universal healthcare and guaranteed medical treatments are the emergency rooms. Unfortunately, these are also the most expensive and the least able to provide continuity of care or adequate follow-up.

Some Uninsured Patients are Afraid to See a Doctor in an Emergency

Then there are the uninsured patients who refuse to use the emergency room regardless. One day when I was on call for my group practice I heard from forty-year-old Barbara, who had suffered a severe coughing spell and lost consciousness. Paramedics rushed to her home, only to find a now conscious Barbara refusing an emergency room evaluation.

She called me later for further advice, explaining she had no insurance. Because she could not afford the emergency room costs, she had sent the paramedics away in distress. Everyone knows about ambulance chasers, but this lady was chasing them away. Barbara was lucky this time but, again for how long? How many others do not go to the emergency room with their serious medical problems because they are uninsured? They are forced to play Russian roulette with their health, their families and their lives.

Another patient, Anna, a young woman in her thirties, worked full time but had no insurance for many years. She called me complaining of lower abdominal pain, abnormal vaginal bleeding and a fever. These symptoms are suggestive of possible serious conditions, such as a tubal pregnancy or a pelvic infection. I insisted she come into the office for an examination and further evaluation.

Initially Anna refused stating, "I have no insurance." I told her that it was necessary that she be seen and not ignore these serious symptoms. Unfortunately, for many uninsured Americans, financial concerns cloud their judgment and place their health in jeopardy.

I was able to persuade her to come into the office. Fortunately for Anna, she did not have a serious problem, but what if she had and hadn't been seen?

Aggravated Hypertension

I met Roy, another strong-bodied, self-employed farmer, for the first time in the emergency room, when he arrived unconscious, having suffered from a severe stroke. His blood pressure was so high that he had bled in his brain. He was only sixty-two years old and uninsured. This was not Roy's first encounter with the emergency room. Five months earlier he had arrived with a badly cut finger; his blood pressure at that time was discovered to be 220/119. (Normal is under 140/90.) The ER doctors sewed up his finger and advised him to follow up with his regular doctor who had been treating his blood pressure. He did see his physician afterwards and blood pressure medication was prescribed.

But now he needed more than just stitches. His current condition required life-support machines, intravenous medications and specialists. It was too late for Roy. His family and doctors had to make the heart wrenching decision to withdraw life support. His chance of regaining any meaningful recovery or even consciousness was lost with the massive stroke. He died three days after admission to the hospital, similar to my patient Emily.

What had happened to Roy between the first emergency room encounter for his cut finger and his last? I spoke with his personal physician about prior treatments and medications. Roy's blood pressure was controlled during the last office visit three months earlier. But he had trouble paying for his prescriptions. He had asked for less expensive blood pressure medications, and the physician did make some changes in treatment. The doctor also remembered that Roy had complained about the costs of some diagnostic tests performed two years earlier. He was still trying to pay those overdue bills.

Affordable medications and health insurance could have made a critical difference in Roy's life. There is no question that delayed or intermittent treatment of high blood pressure leads to premature death from strokes and other diseases. The self-employed frequently go uncovered in a system that primarily depends on employer-based health insurance.

Severe Clinical Depression and More

Joe and his wife Susan, a couple with grown children, came into my office concerned that Susan was severely depressed with suicidal thoughts. I evaluated her potentially life-threatening problem and advised a treatment plan including medications. I thought Joe had come as emotional support and didn't know he needed treatment for medical problems as well. After I had completed her visit, she said, "And one more thing doctor, we have no insurance." Both had been working for their entire adult lives, and Susan had been with the same employer for over twenty years. After all that time, she was still without medical insurance. I gave her some drug samples, scheduled a follow-up appointment and asked her to call the office in two weeks to tell me how she was feeling.

"And how can I help your husband?" I asked. Joe had recently changed jobs and was temporarily uninsured. Simply changing jobs had left him without prescription medication coverage for the next few weeks. Susan asked if I could give Joe samples as well to cover him until his drug benefit began. He had a complicated history of prior heart surgery, diabetes, and hypertension and was currently on ten different prescriptions. I tried to meet his needs with samples as best as I could. I hoped nothing serious would happen to him should he run out of his other medications. Joe and Susan thanked me profusely for the samples, yet I knew this was not the answer to their problems.

Unfortunately Joe eventually lost his job and his health insurance too. Susan's employer finally offered health insurance benefits to her and her family but the majority of the costs came from her paycheck. She showed me her one-week pay stub, which she agreed to let me publish in this book. We both laughed out loud at the "take-home" amount, hardly a decent figure for a full-time employee. But she was willing to pay the high cost to cover her husband's needs. Approximately six months later, her employer sold the business and the new owner decided not to provide health insurance benefits. The couple are among the uninsured of America again.

Some leaders in the government and the insurance industry believe increased tax subsides or deductions will provide decent health insurance

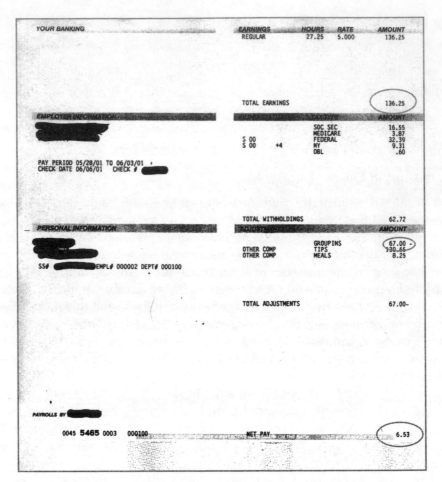

YOUR BANKING				EARNINGS	HOURS	RATE	AMOUNT
				REGULAR	27.25	5.000	136.25
				TOTAL EARNINGS			136.25

EMPLOYER INFORMATION

	FILING STATUS	TAX TYPE	AMOUNT
		SOC SEC	16.55
		MEDICARE	3.87
	S 00	FEDERAL	32.39
	S 00 +4	NY	9.31
		DBL	.60

PAY PERIOD 05/28/01 TO 06/03/01
CHECK DATE 06/06/01 CHECK #

| | | TOTAL WITHHOLDINGS | 62.72 |

PERSONAL INFORMATION

	ADJUSTMENTS		AMOUNT
		GROUP INS	67.00 –
	OTHER COMP	TIPS	130.65
	OTHER COMP	MEALS	8.25

SS#   EMPL# 000002 DEPT# 000100

| | | TOTAL ADJUSTMENTS | 67.00~ |

PAYROLLS BY

0045 **5465** 0003   000100   NET PAY   6.53

Susan's one-week pay stub

coverage to the majority of the uninsured. However, most of the uninsured are low wage earners, children or retirees on fixed incomes. And the average health insurance yearly premium in 1998 for a family in the U.S. was $5,590 (New York State – $6,453) and a single person in the U.S. was $2,176 (New York State – $2,373).[10] Current proposed tax subsides and deductions will cover far less than 50% of the cost of comprehensive insurance for most of the uninsured people in our society who are already struggling to climb out of poverty or even remain in the middle class. Tax deductions would not have helped Joe and Susan, and obviously employer-based health insurance failed them too.

Acute Infection

I met Heather, an assistant manager, in the emergency room when I admitted her for pneumonia. Two years earlier Heather was treated for cancer and osteoporosis-related fractures. She had worked full time for many years, but had no medical insurance. "Only managers get health insurance at my work," Heather told me. She could not afford to see a doctor or pay for health insurance, as she was still paying hospital and doctor bills from two years earlier. One doctor had sent her unpaid bills to a collection agency. Heather said, "I don't even know what he looks like." She commented about the other doctor, "He is really nice and I pay him a little at a time." On this emergency room visit I admitted her to the hospital with an infection for which she had delayed seeking treatment.

Her symptoms had persisted for many weeks, but she had not seen a doctor. If she had been seen earlier as an outpatient and treated with medications, I know this hospitalization could have been avoided. When Heather was discharged, I gave her the "free samples" from my office, but I doubt she will follow up and get the necessary cancer screening tests I recommended. If she returns to the emergency room with a hip fracture or metastatic breast cancer, how much will that cost?

Fractured Ribs

Part time or full time, what is the actual difference, and how do employers define either? Recently I saw Judd, who worked part time for thirty-five hours a week, but had no insurance through his employer. His employer, he told me, only insured "full-time" employees. He had fractured his ribs, and I recommended that he get an x-ray, but he refused. Having no health insurance, Judd was worried about the cost. In most OECD countries and even in some companies in the United States, thirty-five hours a week is considered full time. The United States leads the world in average annual hours worked at 1,966 hours per worker year in 1997. Japan is second at 1,889 hours per worker year, and Great Britain is third at 1,731.[11] Judd was risking further damage; I hope not to a lung.

Chronic Hypertension and Diabetes

Lois was a middle-aged health aid who worked part time for many years at a for-profit or "investor-owned" nursing home. She had a career in the health industry, yet was uninsured and could not afford doctor visits or her prescriptions. It is incredible to me that any health industry employer would deny health insurance benefits to its employees. There is no employer in the healthcare profession who does not know the risks and consequences employees face if they are uninsured. Some employers I know consider health insurance to be too expensive and potentially a penalty to their company's profits. However, I believe companies may benefit if they would invest in the health of their employees. Healthy employees are more productive and may enhance company profits.

Part-time employees are much less likely to be insured than full-time employees. Lois told me that she tried to obtain Medicaid and was turned down because her family's yearly income of $12,200 was too high. Lois suffers from chronic high blood pressure and diabetes, but without health insurance, she did not see her physician for over a year. Having had trouble affording her medications, she went without some. She told me, "I borrowed insulin from my sister who has insurance." Lois had stopped working one year earlier, explaining that she hadn't felt well and couldn't see. Her son's old toy binoculars soon became her means of watching TV. I wondered how she could inject herself with insulin.

No one was surprised when Lois was later admitted to the intensive care unit with a major stroke, severe hypertension and uncontrolled diabetes. Incredibly, she had even stayed at home for three days with her stroke symptoms before coming to the emergency room. Maybe she thought the symptoms would go away. To me, this delay again exemplifies the often unnoticed and unmentioned underclass of uninsured Americans who stand in an interminable "waiting line" for healthcare in this country. The following day, after considerable improvement, she thanked me for not "yelling" at her. Obviously she was feeling guilty for "noncompliance," but how was she to comply? I admit that I may have "yelled" at a similar patient, years earlier, but I have gained more understanding of the human predicament in our country.

I saw Lois in the office after her discharge from the hospital, and she was now compliant, checking her sugars and taking her medications. Sadly however, she had not qualified for Medicaid yet. Her husband still made "too much money," $100 per month over the minimum Medicaid threshold. Her monthly medications easily cost more than that. Her husband said to me, "We have worked all our lives, and we have never asked for handouts. Now we need help and can't get it." Her son thanked me for helping his mother. He told me how he had sent money to her for her prescriptions, but she spent it on food and rent.

Unfortunately, Lois' lack of insurance and her sporadic treatment for diabetes contributed to her inability to work more than a year earlier. Now unable to work or even see, she deals with the physical impairments and suffers. I am certain that her hypertension and elevated cholesterol were also under treated.

There are estimates of the number of people between the ages of eighteen and sixty-five with various diseases who are uninsured for at least one entire year: 528,000 with diabetes, 1.8 million with high blood pressure, and 1.5 million with high cholesterol.[12] How many preventable disabling strokes will other doctors treat next year? How many will I treat? One is too many.

Months later, Lois finally did qualify for Medicaid and was seen by an eye specialist. Her diabetes is now under better control, and her eye specialist eventually operated on her cataracts. I know that her lack of affordable healthcare significantly affected her overall health and contributed to her inability to be gainfully employed. For many years Lois contributed to society. Now she is an early long-term cost. I doubt that she ever will return to even part-time work.

The Working Welfare Mother Syndrome

My wife, also a physician, told me about her patient who refused an x-ray because of no insurance. This patient was previously on Medicaid, but was now a working mother. Working part time at twenty-nine hours per week, she was now making too much money to qualify for Medicaid, leaving her uninsured. Health insurance was only offered to full-time employees, defined as thirty hours or more per week, by this employer. With welfare reform in the late 1990s, many women lost their Medicaid coverage as a consequence of employment. Currently one-third of all working women previously on Medicaid are now uninsured, as are one out of four of their children.[13] Does this consequence of welfare reform make any sense?

I've seen patients lose their insurance as a result of job changes, unemployment, new employment, a move from full to part-time employment, retirement, a family member's death, decisions by employers to drop coverage altogether, and simply the employer's or employee's inability to afford continued insurance premiums. Unfortunately, employer-based health insurance is failing to cover millions of Americans continuously even during record low unemployment and with the largest work force in U.S. history. By 1999 only 55% of all U.S. private sector businesses offered health insurance to their employees with Hawaii being the highest at 83%. New York State private businesses could only manage to offer health insurance to 58% of their employees.[14]

Even Working Aged Adults Need the ICU

I recently spoke at a Continuing Medical Education (CME) conference for doctors about the problems in our current healthcare system. During my presentation, one physician stated quite positively that the number of uninsured people in the U.S. for more than one year in duration was "only 19%" of the total uninsured population. If that were true, then supposedly we may be comforted by the fact that only 8 million of our citizens, the population of New York City, have been without insurance for more than one year. The numbers actually are much greater, as 69% of the uninsured face this dangerous situation for more than a year.[15] This number of people, 30 million, is more than the population of the state of California.

For some people, even healthcare professionals, it's easy to trivialize the problems of the uninsured, and claim that there are only a small number of these human beings. In our local rural community, only 8,000 people are uninsured for more than one year.[16] I just happened to admit two of them to the hospital the night before my CME presentation. Both of these patients were employed full time, but had no doctor and no health insurance.

The first patient, Mike, had risk factors for premature heart disease and had been having chest pains for over three weeks. I admitted him to the cardiac unit in the hospital and "ruled out" a myocardial infarction. However, Mike had an abnormal stress test the following morning and required transfer to a major center for a heart catheterization. Access to a doctor previously could have prevented this expensive hospitalization, emergency transfer and the procedure.

The second uninsured patient of the evening, a young woman named Jennifer, presented to the emergency room by ambulance in a coma from an attempted suicide. She was nearly successful. Luckily, a friend called the paramedics after finding Jennifer unresponsive with empty pill bottles. Later, Jennifer explained how she was depressed for over three months, but had not sought medical or psychiatric help. She had no health insurance and couldn't afford to see a doctor. The empty pill bottles were from her sister's medications. When I asked Jennifer how long she had been uninsured, she responded, "FOREVER!"

Young, adult, white females are the most likely to attempt suicide in America. Elderly, white men are the most successful. You will find three stories in Chapter Nine.

I mention these two patients because they represent the serious illnesses even young adult "healthy" Americans can face. Uninsured patients, regardless of their age, frequently have difficulty in obtaining timely access to medical care in United States.

George the Carpenter

Some uninsured patients suffer many of the signs and symptoms of the illness afflicting the American healthcare system. One such case is that of a fifty-eight year old carpenter named George whom I met in the emergency room seven years ago. He had no previous personal physician and for months had delayed seeking care for a variety of serious symptoms, including blood in his urine and elevated blood sugars. He was self-employed, but unable to afford health insurance given his low and fluctuating income. Even if his income had been higher, there were still the standard clauses barring those with known preexisting medical conditions. So George went without insurance. Even with a severe disease like diabetes he wouldn't see doctors or take medications because of the excessive cost. As is so often the case, denial of his own medical problems and their consequences probably also entered his thinking. The carpenter believed he was "too young" to get sick. Unfortunately, the blood in his urine was from cancer and required major surgery. George, however, was a proud man and knew he could not afford it. He had always paid his bills before, and so he decided to delay his surgery. Apparently he also had a new job for the past eleven weeks and he needed to work one more week to possibly qualify for health insurance benefits. He elected to leave the hospital after a five day stay, forgoing surgery, but promised to come back once insured. I remember wondering how long that would take, and hoped the tumor would not grow any larger.

Regrettably, George failed to return for any office visits or surgery until four months later. When he arrived in the emergency room this time it was for a bloody thumb and not for bloody urine. He accidentally cut off most of his thumb while performing carpentry duties and required emergency surgery. Not surprisingly, we found his diabetes uncontrolled and the tumor larger. The carpenter now agreed to have the cancer surgery, since he was unable to work with a hand injury. Thankfully, he survived the fifteen-day hospital stay, but was now unemployed, disabled and impoverished. He reapplied for Medicaid and found insurance coverage, including medications for his diabetes. He even kept a couple of office visit appointments with me afterwards.

As with many uninsured patients, he only sought medical care when it was an emergency, and as is often the case for the uninsured, the medical bills began to pile up. Prior medical debts accumulated and some of his accounts were sent to a collection agency. One account was for $29 and another was for $281. I'm sure George had others from the first hospitalization.

That was the last time I saw or heard from him until the next emergency nearly one and one-half years later. I wonder if doctors and other health providers realize the consequences of sending patients' bills to collection agencies. I now realize patients who are unable to pay collection notices will not seek timely medical care in the future. Is that the motive of the health providers in the United States? It surely is the effect. I know patients receive different medical care when they have no insurance and lack financial resources versus those patients with "good" insurance or unlimited financial means. This carpenter did not return for his diabetes care, cancer follow-up or other treatments because of the costs and his mounting debt.

When George's thumb healed, he returned to work becoming too "wealthy" for Medicaid again. He had an income and some pensions from prior employment. And he still was too young for Medicare. He rejoined the ranks of the millions of other Americans who are working and uninsured. During these times he would take his medications when he could afford them, and would not take them when he could not.

One year later George faced another emergency, uncontrolled blood sugars and an infected toe. The specialists performed "expensive" tests for him, more procedures and a "minor" amputation. Another eleven days in the hospital for this uninsured diabetic. He re-qualified for Medicaid after this hospitalization and continued to see me in my office as an outpatient. The antibiotics and other medications were now covered for him. But it was too late. The years of under-treated diabetes and vascular disease had caught up to this carpenter. Four months later he had three of his toes removed for a non-healing foot ulcer. This time it was only one day in the hospital. He kept one office appointment but failed to show over the next two years. I received requests for disability information, but I knew he would not qualify yet!

It was two years later and another emergency surgery was needed. This time he presented with vomiting, an elevated blood sugar and an infected gallbladder. During George's medical markedly evaluation we also found a new tumor in his urinary bladder. Routine follow-up cancer screening tests by the specialist would have found his tumor much sooner. Typically, cancer patients, especially those with insurance, undergo routine regular cancer check-ups for years. Their doctors look for evidence of recurrent or possibly new cancers. My patient, on the other hand, had no continuous insurance and couldn't afford to see his doctors. More surgeries and twenty-three hospital days later, the chronically uninsured and under-treated diabetic cancer survivor required another major organ removal.

With his health rapidly failing, and now unable to work, he became impoverished. He was forced to rely on family or friends for shelter, food and medications, because he still didn't qualify for public assistance. Later that year, his kidneys and vision failed and he was unable to care even for his basic needs. Many times his sister found him at home lying on the floor or in bed too weak to stand up. During the next four months he had two more hospitalizations, twelve days total, three ER, two office and multiple home nursing visits to try and control his failing medical condition.

The government finally gave in though, granting him "permanent" Medicaid coverage and they even backdated the coverage four additional months. But his previously under-treated medical problems did not roll back. The carpenter's kidney function deteriorated further, as did his vision. Early detection and/or intervention most likely would have prevented these major surgeries and the attendant expenses. His family never will know how George's course of illness could have been different with "normal" continuous treatment and insurance. Access to suitable healthcare at an earlier period would have made an enormous difference in his life.

The picture of the man on the cover of this book reminds me of George during his illness. I remember him coming to the office unshaven, weak and chronically ill. After his stroke he even had to walk with a walker. The subscript under this picture from the 12th century read, "With rare access to formalized medical care, most people in the Middle Ages relied on folk-healers and, when necessary, devices such as primitive crutches."[18] Not much has changed in healthcare over the centuries for some patients, even those living in the United States.

These true stories demonstrate how the uninsured show up in our emergency rooms suffering the consequences of delayed access to care for serious conditions. Some of these uninsured patients have no regular physician and use the emergency room for their ongoing care. This is probably a more expensive choice of healthcare provider and definitely lacks significant continuity. Other patients delay seeking care because of the cost and fear of mounting medical bills. Unfortunately, I see them wait too long, sometimes needlessly suffering additional morbidity and mortality. Frequently, these additional problems could have been avoided or lessened with earlier treatment. For anyone who still does not believe that lack of health insurance is dangerous in the United States, I suggest reviewing figures one, two and three on pages eighteen and nineteen.

There is also a key issue of justice and humanity, as well as an issue of cost. Many of these stories conclude with treatments that are probably more expensive than prevention. The terrible outcomes only lead to further costs. Families drop into public assistance; welfare picks up nursing home costs; loved ones are lost; family structures are destabilized; children lose love and care. In human terms, the cost of being uninsured is staggering. Why do all of the other OECD nations provide universal care? Most likely they know it is less expensive to prevent diseases than to treat them. All Americans share in paying the costs of the human tragedy of our current healthcare system.

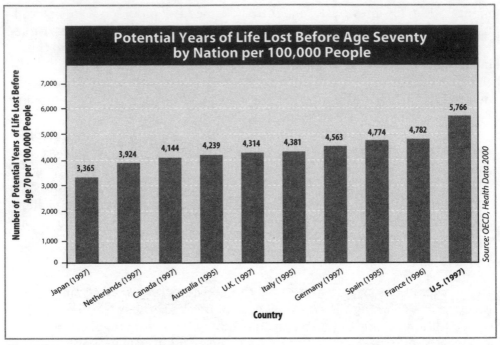

Figure One

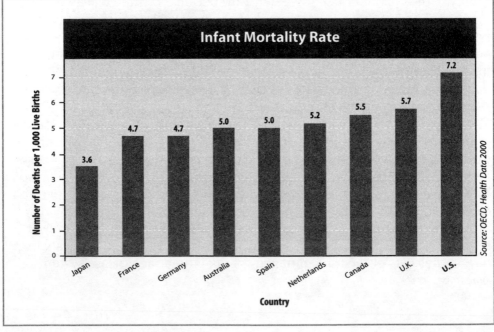

Figure Two

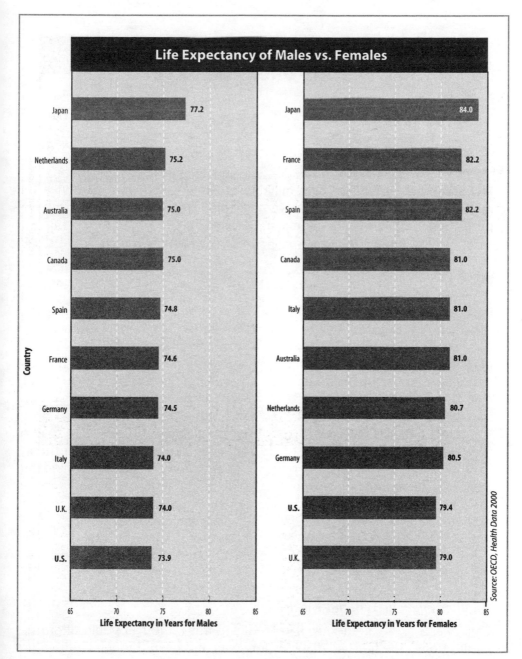

Figure Three

2: THE UNDERINSURED

"The time has arrived to help millions of Americans living without a full measure of opportunity to achieve and enjoy good health...and [to have] protection... against economic effects of sickness."

Harry S. Truman, Sept. 19, 1945

Based on a study of unmet medical needs, the number of underinsured Americans is approximately 42 million, similar to the number of uninsured.[1] Over 90 million Americans lack dental insurance and more than 40% of all Medicare patients lack any outpatient prescription coverage.[2] And, the vast majority of Americans lack long-term insurance.[3] The OECD estimates only 45% of all people in the U.S. are guaranteed comprehensive health insurance coverage comparable to OECD standards.[4]

Underinsured patients have insurance, but they still can't afford all of their needed prescriptions, tests, doctor visits, or hospital bills. In theory, health insurance was meant to protect patients from the economic hardship of sickness. Patients or "consumers" also obtain health insurance to improve their own health. Research and my experience indicate that not all entities of the insurance industry are clear and forthright about their services. Some plans have unaffordable high deductibles or co-pays; some plans fail to cover important medical tests and treatments; and some plans use fine print too small to read in their contracts.

Another Diabetic Without Medication

Carmella, a gray-haired lady, had Medicare but no longer could afford her medications. She has had diabetes for years and been through heart failure and arrhythmias. Recently, we treated her with a blood thinner to prevent a stroke. A specialist also performed an outpatient procedure successfully returning her heart to a normal rhythm. However, she required an expensive medication to maintain this stable condition. Carmella did well until she could no longer afford the expensive medication and stopped taking it.

For two weeks Carmella went without the drug and applied for EPIC, Elderly Pharmaceutical Insurance Coverage, a New York State subsidized prescription plan for low-income elderly persons. During this two-week period, she lapsed back into the arrhythmia. Now she required more blood thinners, other medication changes and another specialist's appointment. I hoped these medication changes would prevent a stroke or worsening heart failure. I know affordable prescriptions for Carmella would have stopped the escalating treatments and costs, and maintained her health.

Over a month later, on a routine phone call to her about her blood thinners, I asked, "What did the specialist say?" She responded, "They wouldn't see me until I paid up my bill, $158."

I couldn't believe it and said, "You have to see them." Again she responded," I am doing the best I can. I can't afford to see the doctor." I called the specialist's office. An administrator told me the patient had been sent to collections twice in the past and had not paid her deductible. I insisted they see her for another outpatient procedure. They eventually agreed, because I "asked." What would have happened to Carmella if I had not intervened?

When she eventually did see the specialist for the procedure, her blood pressure was too low. Now she required a four-day hospital stay for medication adjustments and intravenous fluids. Her specialist and I knew this hospitalization could have been prevented with affordable medications for Carmella. Does Medicare or any other health insurer really save money or lives by not providing affordable prescription coverage to all of their patients? I very much doubt they do.

Heart Failure, Coronary Artery Disease, Hypertension, and Diabetes

One of my long-time patients, Darlene, came into my office in tears. She was severely ill after she had stopped taking her medications for heart failure, diabetes, coronary disease and high blood pressure. She had Medicare and had invested in a $10,000 lifetime limit prescription drug insurance policy. She had "used up" her drug limit with her multiple medications. Then she started to use her credit cards to buy her medications, but as she said, "got in trouble." The credit card interest alone took its toll. So then she "went without" her medications for nearly two months. When I saw her in the office, she had lost twenty pounds, had a blood sugar over 600 (normal is below 126), heart failure and chest pains.

"Why haven't I seen you for the past year?" I questioned. "I was feeling so good," Darlene said. "You know that I baby sit these kids. I take care of them while their mother is at work. I get them on and off the school bus. It's better than sitting at home in my rocking chair all day!" she chokingly mentioned as tears rolled down her cheeks.

I questioned further, "Why didn't you ask your family for help?" "They have their own problems and I didn't want to bother them. It hurts my pride to ask for help," Darlene explained as she hung her head in shame.

I later admitted her to the ICU and a five-day hospital stay. I'm sure that Darlene's hospitalization cost Medicare more than her entire medication costs in the past decade. I gave her multiple samples at the time of the hospital discharge, while her son helped her enroll in EPIC.

Thankfully, her health recovered and she didn't have a heart attack. She returned to doing the things she loved, caring for those children. Recently though, on a routine follow-up visit, she said, "Should I have my cataract surgery done?" I asked, "How's your vision?" "Not too good. Everything is in a fog, a haze," she said. I explained that she should have it done then. But she wanted to know if surgery three months from now was too long a wait.

"I thought they only had waiting lines in Canada!" I joked. Darlene quickly fired back, "It took me another three months to get the appointment in the first place." I then watched her try to read some medication changes I had written down for her on a piece of paper. She held it less than six inches from her face. How can I expect her to manage at home with her diabetes equipment and medications?

Diabetes Too Soon

I saw another diabetic with the same drug insurance coverage as Darlene. She, too, had a lifetime limit of $10,000 for her medications. I advised her to start some new medication for her uncontrolled diabetes. However, she refused because she didn't want to deplete her insurance plan "too soon." She wanted to save her insurance policy for the future. I couldn't convince her that controlling her diabetes now was extremely important to her future health. There is no question that patients place their health at risk because of the financing choices they must make while trying to cope with being underinsured. It is sad; it is tragic; and it wouldn't happen if they lived in Europe, Japan, or Canada.

An Out-of-State Visitor

I hospitalized Harry, who was visiting from another state. He told me he suddenly stopped his medications prior to this hospitalization, "Too many pills and too much money; over $500 a month." Harry required admission to the hospital because of his trouble breathing, heart failure and chronic leukemia. When I placed him back on his usual medications, he improved and was discharged home. This hospitalization alone cost more than a two year supply of his chronic medciations.

A Metastic Cancer Survivor

I have cared for Moira, a lovely lady, for years now. She is fast approaching ninety-two years of age. We diagnosed a metastatic cancer years earlier after she presented with a bowel obstruction. There was no effective treatment for this type of tumor and so I prescribed large doses of narcotics to control her pain. Unfortunately they were very expensive. Sadly during this same time period she lost two sons from sudden illness and she herself nearly went without pain medications.

One day she told me that she was considering stopping her $430 per month regime of narcotics because she was running out of money. She then explained how she had won a legal settlement from a previous injury due to a fall and was able to continue paying for her pain medications with her settlement funds. How many different ways do patients in the United States have to obtain the financial resources to afford their medications?

Another Well-Off Senior

An elderly lady, Harriet, came in the office wheezing and short of breath. I prescribed some medication, but she said she couldn't afford to fill them at the pharmacy for two weeks. She didn't have the money. Previously she had a Medicare HMO with premiums of $83 per month and $10 prescription co-pay charges. She changed her coverage to a $50 per month premium, but now her drug plan covered only $500 yearly on the first $1,000 spent. Here is another example of how the insurance industry has shifted the high cost of medications onto the seniors.

If Harriet ends up in the ER or hospital with a delayed treatment for bronchitis, how exactly did any money get saved? And despite what others may think, the elderly are not "well off" in the United States. In 1997, they spent 23% of their income on out-of-pocket expenses for healthcare.[5] That only includes the elderly people who actually received the care. It is a good question as to what the figure would have been if all elderly patients were actually able to pay for all the health services they needed.

Chronic Psychiatric Illness; A Long Bus Ride

I was consulted concerning a patient named Cliff at the alcohol rehabilitation inpatient program in Jamestown, New York. A man in his forties, Cliff required hospitalization for treatment of his chronic psychiatric illness, alcoholism and drug abuse. Since Cliff lived in a large city in New York all his life, I asked him how he found his way to our hospital in Jamestown. He said, "Your hospital was the nearest hospital in the state that would treat my multiple problems."

I started to laugh; I knew this was another sick story. His hometown is much larger than Jamestown and many hours away by bus. In New York State, very few hospitals are farther away from his hometown than our hospital.

Cliff proceeded to tell me what had happened. He was diagnosed with a psychiatric disorder over twenty years ago, and had been under a psychiatrist's care in his hometown. He was treated with two and sometimes three different medications and saw the same psychiatrist for many years. He also had abused drugs or alcohol intermittently during this period of his life. But, he was able to maintain employment with the same company for eighteen years and had health insurance. He actually did his job well and made a decent living wage of $40,000-$50,000 per year. In the 1990s, he had major surgery after which he took four more medications every day.

Some years later, Cliff's life changed again. He admitted he made some poor choices, including abusing alcohol and cocaine. His company laid him off because of "downsizing." I believe it was more likely related to his health problems.

He told me, "My bosses would go out and drink at lunch time, but it was not OK for me to drink."

Even though he was unemployed and financially strapped, he continued seeing his psychiatrist. The patient even maintained his insurance through "COBRA" over the next six months. But the medical bills began to mount up. "I paid $1,500 of my severance pay to the doctor," he told me. "Why $1,500?" I asked.

Cliff explained how his insurance was "not enough" after only partially covering his psychiatric care. The insurance paid $35 per doctor office visit, while his co-pay was another $25. Having weekly psychiatric office visits added up over time. In addition, Cliff still had to pay monthly insurance premiums. He told me how the psychiatrist once reminded him of his outstanding bill during an emergency room visit.

In America, market forces have increasingly failed psychiatric patients. Mental health coverage by private insurance has been falling steadily over the past few years. Of the total insurance premiums paid in 1998, only 3% went towards mental health services, a 55% reduction over the previous ten years.[6] At the same time, patients are faced with higher and higher co-pays for mental health services. One large managed care program in Ohio consumed over 45% of the mental health insurance premium on overhead and profits. While at the same time, the mental health program failed to supply any providers in some of the "covered" counties.[7]

When Cliff lost his long-term employment, he explained how he found low paying jobs at the local restaurants but was offered no health insurance benefits. "Only managers had health insurance," he explained. How often I have heard that. Now financially stressed and unable to afford the insurance payments, Cliff went without health insurance. His doctors gave him samples to the best of their ability. Soon he stopped taking his non-psychiatric medications altogether and cut back on his psychiatric appointments "I felt so wrong seeing the psychiatrist without paying him," Cliff admitted. "Why not apply for Medicaid?" I questioned. Cliff said, "I made too much money, over $340 per month."

And here is what happens to many psychiatric patients without adequate insurance and affordable treatment. Four months later Cliff was homeless, off prescription medication, and destitute. He checked into a mission in his hometown. The counselor recommended he "file for bankruptcy, quit his restaurant jobs, and then apply for Medicaid." He did that and he finally qualified for Medicaid. He received help for his alcoholism; however, the counselor felt he needed long-term drug and alcohol treatment, plus psychiatric care. The mission told him our Jamestown hospital was "the closest hospital in New York State" that could treat his multiple illnesses, psychiatric, drug and alcohol problems.

I asked the nurse, "How did he get here?"

"They gave him a bus ticket and sent him here," she explained.

"Was it a one or two-way ticket?" I asked.

"A two-way ticket," the nurse responded. I thought maybe someone hoped he would lose the return ticket or wander into Pennsylvania. "We have been getting a lot of these referrals recently," she added.

With proper health insurance all along, Cliff would have been treated in his own hometown under his own doctor's care, and possibly avoided hospitalization, hopelessness and homelessness in the first place. He had not committed any crimes that I am aware of, other than probably possession of cocaine. But, how many people with untreated mental illness, drug abuse, or alcoholism commit crimes and become imprisoned, or descend into homelessness? The costs to society in both economic and human terms are enormous. America had nearly 2,000 jails and prisons in 1998, a 600% increase over the previous twenty-five years.[8]

A Loner

An elderly patient, Sarah, lived alone and frequently refused any home care offered. She was a very proud, but angry woman, suspicious of anyone who tried to help. As her illness progressed, she weakened and was no longer able to transfer from bed to chair alone. With this she became more receptive to home care and our help. Unfortunately, Sarah couldn't afford to hire home health aides and her Medicare provided only minimal amounts of home care per week. When I saw she was unable to manage at home alone, I hospitalized her and requested a nursing home. She initially refused the nursing home, but after much persuasion from the family, the nurses and myself, she eventually agreed.

However, the nursing home refused to accept Sarah until she qualified for Medicaid. Medicaid denied coverage until it investigated an $8,000 recent withdrawal from her checking account. So Sarah remained in the hospital forty-one days before final approval and acceptance. The cost of this prolonged hospital stay was far more than the disputed $8,000 withdrawal. She probably could have avoided the hospitalization entirely and remained at home if more home health services were available to her, but it was too expensive. The American healthcare system wasted forty-one days of hospitalization and put her in a nursing home at significant multiples of the cost of home care.

A "Lucky" Veteran

A fifty-seven year old man, Brian, has severe multiple sclerosis and has been wheelchair dependent for several years. He was a veteran who fought in Vietnam and later worked for another government agency. Now with this devastating illness, Brian was unable to transfer, walk or bathe himself. But his family and aides were wonderful and took very good care of him. His skin was in great condition; he never had any bedsores.

The other day I asked how the family was able to manage him. Brian currently receives twenty hours a week of home health aides paid for by the VA. His father, he told me, had "to fight" for more assistance from the Veterans Administration (VA) to increase the home help from ten to twenty hours per week. Surprisingly, Brian could pay for the rest of his home care if the family couldn't. The VA also told him that if he needs more home care, then it's "the nursing home."

From his wheelchair Brian told me he was "lucky" to get twenty hours per week of home aid. How was he "lucky" when he was the one in the wheelchair? And what happens to the patient who doesn't have a supportive family or the financial resources? Is it "the nursing home" or premature death? What is the rationale of that? Forty hours of home care is far less than the cost of a nursing home, and what about Brian who wanted to be with his loving family?

A Mother With Dementia

Dementia is a common problem for the aging population. Some estimates predict 20% of people over eighty and 50% of those over ninety years old, will have dementia.[9] In my practice, dementia accounts for one-third of all nursing home patient placements. One elderly patient, Blanche, had moderately severe dementia and was cared for at an adult group home, which is less expensive than a nursing home. Her other health problems included heart failure, prior strokes, and arrhythmias. She, too, didn't have prescription (Rx) coverage. Because of her dementia, Blanche was unable to make decisions for herself. Her son, having the power of attorney (POA), would not apply for Rx assistance through Medicaid or EPIC. I'm not sure why.

One day I received a phone call from the adult group home manager. He was concerned over their resident, Blanche. The pharmacy would no longer deliver her medications because the POA had not paid the Rx bill. The manager asked for my assistance, "Do you have samples or could you call the son?" Adult protection was also contacted. The money came through and the pharmacy delivered the Rxs. But has the problem been solved? Just recently this same situation recurred and required the same intervention. I'm sure that Blanche would qualify for either EPIC or Medicaid, if only she were mentally capable of filing an application. In most other wealthy nations of the world, she would not have to file such applications for prescription coverage.

A Work-Related Injury to a Diabetic

Tim, a veteran who had served his country well, had been working full time with health and worker's compensation insurance. But because of a job-related injury the previous year, he was forced to leave his employment. Seven months later, he couldn't afford his insurance for himself or his family and also provide food, housing and clothing. Tim's worries grew as his family was now also uninsured.

For many months prior to his first emergency room visit with me, Tim experienced symptoms of high blood sugars. He would not see his regular doctor without health insurance, but he would see his worker's compensation doctor for his injury. He received treatment for the injury, but no evaluation or treatment for the elevated sugars. Then one weekend, after severe confusion, hallucinations and profound weight loss, his wife brought him to the emergency room. His blood sugar was over 2,000. The number "2,000" is not a typographical error, a normal blood sugar is less than 126. He had multiple medical problems, extreme dehydration, electrolyte imbalances and chest pain. He was hospitalized for six days; several were spent in the intensive care unit.

Miraculously, Tim survived this illness and eventually went home after being given "free samples" from our office. Hopefully, they would hold him over until he possibly qualified for Medicaid or VA services. When we talked about why he procrastinated in seeking care, he said, "The first fifteen years we were married, we had no insurance and we learned to get by without. If my wife or children got sick, they'd see the doctor, maybe. If I got sick, I learned to live with it. One time I broke my hand and couldn't use it for a while. It costs money to get it fixed and I didn't want the bills." "What would you have done about this illness if you had insurance?" I pondered. He said, "I would have come in sooner, but 'IF' is a big word."

A Mother's Story

An elderly patient of mine, Corrine, told me how her son, Paul, recently had died from massive bleeding after a ruptured aneurysm. I asked her, "Who was his doctor?" She went on to tell me that he didn't have a doctor. He apparently had endured chest and back pains for many months. Again, another example of the waiting lines many people in America face. She told me many more sad facs about his life. I asked her if she would write her son's story for this book and she agreed. "I've always wanted to write a book," she said. Here is what she sent:

> Our son Paul was a brilliant electrical engineer, who left college to serve in the military. He completed his tour with honors, over and beyond the call of duty. He was a young man in a hurry, who met every challenge in the corporate world for thirty-six years. Along the way he encountered all the intrigue, greed and politics that go with big business. One day at the peak of his career, he was asked to rule and pass on something that, if there were an accident, could have caused many people to be killed. Negotiations came to a standstill. Paul refused and walked away from a six-figure income with all its perks. He would not compromise his integrity, which was well known around the world.
>
> He had married his childhood sweetheart, who came to the marriage with an alcohol problem from her youth. This became more apparent as the years went on. They had a beautiful home, three lovely children and four grandchildren.
>
> My son suffered years of illness, several cancer operations and rehabilitation. The expenses mounted. The stress of work and worry over his family began to take its toll. He never got around to taking care of himself, even though the coverage for medical care was there. Then came a time when no insurance was available and he went bankrupt.
>
> His wife could not handle that and left to go to live with her

daughter. She opted for a separation, thinking that he would return to his previous work and health. Paul finally opted for divorce and then returned home to us. We never realized what his life had been.

He said, "I came back home to spend whatever days we all have left to spend with you, Dad and Marie Ellen," his sister. We all experienced a great sadness at that time.

He spent hours talking with his sister. The bond between them has always been very close. His dad and I talked to him about his work and the things we had done together and our plans for the future. We all looked forward to a new beginning with his great zest for all the new technology waiting to be used. Paul had a great sense of humor and loved repartee. We look back and wonder if the circumstances had been different what could have been.

He had lost a lot of weight during this time and we all succeeded, finally, to get him in to see a doctor. We went to the VA locally and found a doctor he liked very much. He was examined and had an appointment to go back for tests. When he returned for the tests, he found that this doctor was no longer there. As is the custom with any government process, everything takes longer and so there were more delays. Finally, my son tried the VA in Buffalo, but there was still so much delay and red tape that he decided the two-hour, one-way commute was not worth the effort.

When he collapsed at home on Memorial Day weekend, the rescue squad took him to the hospital. A thoracic surgeon and his staff performed a seven-hour operation. They used twenty-four pints of blood and sent for platelets from Buffalo. It was a heroic effort, but too late.

Two days later we said a tearful goodbye. He was a loving and caring son, father and brother. We were all blessed to have had him. He had a military funeral, and his wife received the flag. After taps sounded, his son wearing a tartan bearing his father's medals, played the mournful bagpipes.

Once his country honored him. Now we honor him and what he prized most, "Family and country above all else."

Signed, Corrine, Paul's mother

Corrine also enclosed Paul's obituary but it failed to mention that he died from lack of universal health insurance. He was employed, but he died at the age of sixty-four, just shy of automatic Medicare coverage. He had no locally accessible physician, some VA health insurance, symptoms of back pain for many months, and a sudden, painful death.

His surgery, with over twenty-four units of blood and seven hours in the OR, cost far more than providing him with health insurance when he needed it. In his life story I read how he worked for the airline industry. How many lives did he save with his decision to refuse passage of a design flaw? Affordable, accessible, comprehensive health insurance would have saved this man from bankruptcy, and probably also his life.

A Bankrupt Judge

An elderly patient Judy, a retired judge, had Medicare, but no prescription coverage. She had multiple medical problems including chronic abdominal pain, respiratory distress, arthritis and high blood pressure. She declared bankruptcy after using credit cards to pay for her prescriptions. In 1999, over 45% of all bankruptcies in the U.S. were related to medical reasons or large medical debt. Five men per 1,000 and seven women per 1,000 suffered from a medical-related bankruptcy in 1999.[10]

Judy tried to obtain prescription help and applied for spousal Medicaid, but was turned down because she owned her home. Her husband Daniel, suffering the effects of a stroke and severe arthritis already received Medicaid. Daniel now lives in a crowded nursing home because of his medical problems and Judy's inability to care for him.

Amazingly, if Daniel dies, Judy will then qualify for Medicaid drug benefits. If she had suffered the stroke first, then her husband would have gone broke from his medication costs. For now, she remains in her own home and refused a nursing home herself. Her family tries to care for her basic needs as best as they can.

I stopped asking her to come for office visits. I felt guilty as she would gasp for air just walking into the exam room, something so basic and simple that most people never think about. Sometimes I feared it was her last breath. Now I make house calls and hopefully, make a small difference for her and her family. In her living room hangs a great picture of her, the judge, sitting behind the bench presiding over the court. Some judges have lifetime prescription coverage, but not Judy. Adequate health insurance and prescription coverage could have made an enormous difference in her life. How much of her illness was due to stress and financial strain? Underinsurance can wreak havoc in the middle class, too.

He Failed to Collect Rent

A sixty-one year old man, Milton, worked most of his life and supported his family until he became disabled with severe non-operable coronary artery disease, heart failure, arrhythmia, and uncontrolled diabetes. He continuously runs out of his medications, which are not covered by Medicare. Sometimes I can keep up with his needs with our samples and sometimes not. I don't have some of the medications he needs. Milton frequently arrives in my office or emergency room with uncontrolled heart failure requiring treatment or hospitalization. His hospitalizations have easily cost Medicare many times more than providing him "free" medication insurance coverage. He recently ran out of some medications for two weeks and he doesn't qualify for Medicaid (because he's too wealthy) or EPIC (because he's too young). This time he didn't ask me for samples, perhaps being too embarrassed. Instead, his girlfriend borrowed money to buy his medications.

I later referred Milton to Catholic Charities. They couldn't believe Milton did not qualify for Medicaid. His income was $1,000 per month, but his medication costs were $500 per month. Catholic Charities told me the Medicaid office turned him down because, "He didn't charge his girlfriend rent, $200 per month." I spoke with him about this and he said, "She has lived with me for ten years. Previously she abused drugs and was an alcoholic. I agreed to take her in, if she got off the drugs and alcohol. She has been clean since." America has a sick healthcare system that denies vital prescription coverage to sick patients and denies Medicaid coverage to people helping others.

The more underinsured Milton's needs are, the more expensive his costs are for Americans. The only way society will save money on Milton is if he dies quickly at home.

An Elderly Man

An elderly patient, Jim, called my office for refills on his insulin needles. I had not seen him in over a year and requested that he also come in for an evaluation. When I first met Jim two years ago, he was very sick with uncontrolled diabetes, emphysema and non-operable coronary artery disease. His cardiac catheterization at that time showed only one open artery remaining from his prior heart bypass surgery years earlier. Jim continues to smoke, lives alone and has Medicare, but no medication coverage (He probably would have qualified for EPIC but never applied).

I actually was surprised when he called. I thought that he would have had more health problems since his last visit. He was on multiple medications at the last visit, but now he was only taking insulin and aspirin. When I asked him why he hadn't come into the office sooner or had not continued his Rxs, he stated, "I have to eat, you know!" The choices some patients make are incredible. Jim chose cigarettes, an addictive and harmful drug, over vital medications. But effective smoking cessation therapy is not covered by his insurance plan. What would be more cost effective? Helping someone stop the habit of an addicting drug, or paying for the cancer surgery, or a coronary bypass?

Another patient, an elderly lady on multiple medications said, "I couldn't eat if not for EPIC." We make vulnerable people in our society "sign-up" and prove their "eligibility" for necessary healthcare coverage. I believe this demonstrates another sign and symptom of the massive systemic illness in American healthcare.

Another Prescription Dilemma

An elderly patient, Julia, had prior heart surgery. She also has emphysema, high blood pressure, and arthritis. She missed qualifying for EPIC by $200 a month. As her total income was only $800 a month, and one-half of this went towards her Rx costs of $400 a month, how can she not qualify for a government prescription program?

She told me, "I had better give up some of those medications; they're so expensive." She actually already had stopped some of her prescriptions that I thought were important to maintaining her health. "You have to rob Peter to pay Paul. And that doesn't make Peter happy!" she commented. The sick and elderly frequently have to make difficult decisions between necessary medications and other life necessities. Among the wealthy nations, the United States is the only nation that does not provide nearly universal prescription coverage to its elderly citizens.[11]

A $5,000 Deductible

I asked a patient, Madge, "Why don't you go to the county clinic for your Pap smear and mammogram." The county clinic had provided these services to patients at no charge. Madge responded, "I don't have insurance. Actually I do, but I have a $5,000 per year deductible and it costs me a fortune. In a couple years I'll have insurance when I have Medicare. They raised my deductible from $2,500 to $5,000 last year and I'm still paying the same premiums, $140 per month. And this insurance plan didn't even cover prescriptions."

She agreed to have the mammogram and Pap smear with me when she gained Medicare, but for now refused anymore screening tests I offered. When will we learn how much this delay will cost? It seems like some insurance company is playing games with Madge's wallet and possibly her life.

Another Elderly Patient

An elderly man, Fred, had multiple risk factors for vascular disease and presented with bilateral leg pain and poor pulses in the legs. His pain stopped him from exercising. I advised him to have a non-invasive vascular blood flow test, and possibly an angiogram, to see if he needed further treatment. He declined any of the tests, explaining, "I'll have to pay for it." Fred's insurance had a high deductible and 20% co-payment.

A History of TB

A patient, Erika, had a history of tuberculosis (TB) exposure and continued to smoke cigarettes. I advised her to stop smoking, obtain a screening mammogram and a chest x-ray. She declined, stating, "I haven't met my deductible. I have better places to spend my money." And then, in reference to long-term care, she further replied, "I'm not going to a nursing home. They can take my house, but I'm still not going!"

Medical Savings Accounts

I believe these stories demonstrate significant reasons why Medical Savings Accounts or high deductible insurance plans will fail to deliver the necessary services, therapeutic or preventive, and will eventually reduce the quality of medical care overall, especially for people in lower income brackets or in poor health.

MSA means Medical Saving Accounts, another new American idea to save the nation from the high costs of medical care. Individuals will buy high deductible insurance policies from private companies and place other funds into a savings account for future potential medical costs. I believe these plans will not reduce overall costs in America, but will only increase them. They also will create more potential or real harm for the patients, the people this system is supposedly designed to serve.

Most of the costs for medical care (72%) go to a small percentage of the people (10%).[12] At least 10% of all patients will easily exhaust their savings when they face their expensive illnesses. And many Americans with these high deductible plans will still be beholden to the "for-profit" private insurance industry that needs to make a profit. Quality of medical care will also suffer when MSA patients are required to pay out-of-pocket or use their savings for preventive services. I believe many Americans will delay obtaining necessary preventive services, unfortunately a common occurrence when people have to spend money on their health. Sometimes I think we want vaccines, mammograms, sigmoidoscopies, Pap smears, prostate exams, dental exams and cleanings and even some blood tests to be "free." Patients fear these exams and tests, for they sometimes hurt or deliver potential "bad" news. Making patients pay, especially significant amounts, for these lifesaving tests or treatments will reduce their overall use. This will again lead to more expensive illnesses or premature death, a common occurrence suffered by the underinsured. MSA demonstrates more incremental reforms that will fail to correct the nation's sick health system. This nation's present health system seems to place money and profits ahead of patients, resulting in further harm to many of the patients it supposedly serves.

And do not look to the MSA to reduce bureaucracy, for the insurers will need to keep track of out-of-pocket costs and so will the patients, essentially doubling the record keeping. Even the Congressional Budget Office projected MSA would increase Medicare costs by $2 billion alone.[13]

A Double-Covered Patient

In a move to lower the cost of Medicare, the government has encouraged seniors to join HMOs. One HMO Medicare patient, also a veteran, could not afford his three prescription co-pays in the HMO. The co-pays were "too much." So he went to the VA because the prescriptions were "free." To obtain the VA medications, the double-covered patient had to be examined by a VA primary care doctor. His new doctor ordered more tests and changed his prescriptions to their formulary. The VA physician also found blood in his urine, but did not evaluate the bleeding source. The VA referred the patient back to me. Where are the savings for the federal government with three different programs for this patient? And considering the runaround, the extra tests and medication changes this patient endured, I would hardly call this quality medical care; surely it is not consumer friendly service.

A Traveling Veteran

I do not mean to be disrespectful to the VA or brave veterans who served our country. I was fortunate to have some training in the VA during my internal medicine residency. However, do we not want the best treatment for all Americans, including veterans?

My patient, Vito, had a serious life-threatening infection that required expensive surgery and prolonged antibiotics. An infectious disease specialist from a university hospital initially prescribed the treatment. Vito could not afford this long-term medication costing hundreds of dollars a month, so he tried the VA. Unfortunately, the VA specialist would not approve the drug coverage unless the patient was seen in their VA clinic. This required the patient to travel two hours one-way by automobile while in pain and still recovering from his surgery. Then there was the clinic wait and more tests, but eventually the VA came through for Vito.

I believe tests, doctor visits, and medications are duplicated or changed almost every time dual insured patients use the VA and other providers simultaneously. These changes and duplicities are an added and unnecessary cost for the federal government. Furthermore they greatly increase the chance of medication, treatment and provider errors. Why does this country allow such untoward bureaucracy to continue to fall on the patients, doctors, and hospitals when a universal national health program could eliminate the multitudes of insurance programs and provide quality coverage to all people in this nation?

No Pain Medications, Please

My patient, James, had health insurance but the drug co-pays were too expensive for him. He had many health problems and was on chronic expensive narcotics. He had seen virtually every specialist in town over the past few years. The patient decided to use the VA for his medication coverage. Unfortunately, the VA physician would not authorize a refill on his narcotics and the patient ran out. Four days later, the patient was in severe pain plus narcotic withdrawal and required hospitalization. Not in the VA, though! I am not sure why the patient didn't call me as I would have re-written his medication. I think he couldn't afford them and needed the VA's help.

Later his HMO refused to cover this hospitalization. Not only that, but they also denied a breathing apparatus at home for his documented sleep disorder, sleep apnea. One day while doing rounds, I noticed that James had a sleeping disorder. I ordered a sleep study and the specialist confirmed the diagnosis. The specialist recommended treatment with a breathing apparatus at home, one the patient would wear at night, to prevent the sleep disorder. The specialist and I both ordered the treatment device but James still does not have it. By saving money for the device will the HMO cause a far more expensive hospitalization or do they plan to deny coverage of that too?

A Rare Disease

A patient named Robert presented to the ER with abdominal pain and a chronic mental disorder. His physician was not on staff at our hospital and Robert was a member of a Medicaid HMO. We actually made the diagnosis, a very rare disease. I'd never seen an actual patient with this particular disorder. I talked to his previous physician after discharge and the patient did follow-up with me a couple of times as an outpatient. I had earned the patient's respect during his recent illnesses, but unfortunately I didn't participate in his insurance plan. Later against his wishes, he returned to his original physician. Patients in America often do not have the freedom to choose their personal physician.

Interestingly, during my temporary care for him, he developed a case of bronchitis requiring treatment in the hospital. I advised him to stop smoking and he agreed. He wanted help and so I prescribed the nicotine patch.

He never filled the prescription because he could not afford the out-of-pocket cost of $60 per month for the patches.

"Look!" I said, "At two dollars per pack and a pack a day, that's the cost of the patches."

His girlfriend responded, "He only smokes half a pack."

I replied, "Ok, then that's $30."

Robert then jumped in with a smile and said, "Ten dollars a carton… on the reservation." In a nearby town Seneca Indians sell tax-free cigarettes.

"How do you get there?" I asked.

Robert responded, "On the bus."

"What bus?" I inquired. "The Medicaid bus, it takes me to my dentist appointments in Buffalo." he answered.

Robert further explained how the bus driver stops at the Indian reservation so passengers can buy "tax free" tobacco products or low-cost cigarettes. It seems ironic that a Medicaid-financed bus en route to a Medicaid-financed dentist can stop at a tax-free reservation. And Robert must make this long distance bus ride out-of-town because only two dentists participate with Medicaid in our county.

A "Lucky" Artist?

An eighty-two year old man, Bill, had a stroke and nearly complete paralysis of his left leg. He had failed inexpensive aspirin therapy prior to the stroke. His specialist and I changed his medication to a more expensive blood thinner, which we hoped would prevent another stroke. He was in a Medicare HMO with only partial prescription coverage. His treatment also required another hospitalization and nursing home care for rehabilitation.

Over many months Bill improved considerably and returned home. However, his family recently asked if he could stop using the expensive medication because he was having trouble affording his Rxs. When he came into the office, he told my medical student, "I sold two paintings for $100 each. My hands are still good. I guess I can always sell my paintings for my medications." I suppose he's "lucky" that the stroke only affected his leg.

A Loving Daughter

A loving daughter, Amy, spent $31,000 of her own money on caring for her mother's illness and home healthcare needs. After her mother died, Amy's own health problems worsened and she was running out of money to pay for her own Rxs. She had private health insurance that didn't cover the medication costs. She was depending on her life savings for her own needs in the future, but instead depleted them trying to take care of her mother. Over 85% of the home care needs of the elderly are provided by the patient and family themselves.[14] Amy's mother remained in her own home instead of being shipped off to a nursing home. Amy is not eligible for Medicaid at this time.

Not in Poverty Yet

Mitch, an insulin dependent diabetic patient of nearly fifty years, had trouble obtaining his medications. Disabled with poor vision, his other problems included high blood pressure, high cholesterol and peripheral vascular disease. He wanted to obtain insulin and other supplies from the drug companies at no cost. To complete the "Patient Assistance Program" enrollment application he also included a copy of his Social Security check ($914 per month) plus his insulin and supply costs ($270 per month). When asked why he did not qualify for Medicaid coverage, he wrote "not in poverty yet" twice on the application.

Mitch's enrollment application

Without insulin for even a few days, Mitch would lapse into a coma, require hospitalization or die. How can his $644 monthly income, Social Security minus medication costs, be considered "Not in poverty yet?" In America we have segmented and raised the cost of healthcare to the point where such lines are drawn to prevent people from being healthy.

These are just a few examples of the financial and medical hardships the underinsured patients face in the United States. Does under-insurance affect their health outcomes? Is America really saving any money in "the big picture" with so many insurance companies, state and federal healthcare programs, high co-pays and deductibles, inadequate home care or unapproachable prescription coverage for millions? I doubt it!

Patients can have insurance and still be in "the underclass." They frequently suffer the same as their uninsured brethren. At times they lack basic healthcare, and suffer premature disability, illnesses and even untimely death. The system costs much more than would otherwise be needed with proper preventive and intervention care.

Sadly, President Truman's call over fifty-five years ago for "good health...and protection...against economic effects of sickness," has not been heard for the uninsured and the underinsured in this country. Rather, Truman's initiative may have had an unintended result. It was in response to his proposal that the healthcare industry coalesced into a lobby with the main purpose of avoiding universal coverage and government funding of healthcare. The lobby fears patient equality, public accountability and public administration. The industry has successfully blocked enactment of a universal national health program for over fifty years. In that time, the other industrialized democracies have made decent healthcare a goal that is reachable for every citizen and have financed almost all of their systems from public funding sources.

The United States so-called market-driven system is fundamentally flawed as further evidenced by the experiences of insured patients which will be described in the following chapter.

3: THE INSURED

"It is more honorable to repair a wrong than to persist in it."
Thomas Jefferson, 1806

The last chapter described those who do not have sufficient health insurance for a variety of reasons. Coverage for a little more than half of the insured people and their families, is comprehensive and includes a prescription drug benefit, dental benefits, and low or no out-of-pocket costs. This number is declining, however. For the others, slightly less than half, with their insurance plans or HMOs, there's a question of how much freedom and access to healthcare they really have.

Newspapers and TV reports, reflecting the healthcare lobby perceptions, bemoan the waiting lines, lack of specialty care, rationing and other perceived poor results of nations with universal healthcare. Any call for a national health program meets with the Pavlovian response, "That's socialized medicine!" I'm not sure the public or even doctors know exactly what that means. Hardly anyone rationally advocates "government-run" healthcare in this country. This country's market-driven system is postulated to offer freedom of choice, enormous access and high quality to its patients. The reality, on the other hand, is far different for my patients and the "slightly less than half" of the insured patients. These are the stories of what happens to people with insurance.

Afraid to Use

Most insured Americans receive their coverage through their employer. But, even patients with employer-based insurance sometimes face delays in obtaining necessary healthcare. My patient, Bart, feared he might lose his job if he used his medical insurance. Bart is a diabetic and had experienced heart disease and a prior heart catheterization. When he started having more chest pain, I adjusted his medications and advised him to see a cardiologist and consider another heart catheterization. Bart declined, fearing the tests would cost his insurance company and eventually his employer too much money. He told me he was afraid the added healthcare costs to his employer would eventually lead to his losing his job. He explained, "I can't lose my job; I only have one and a half more years to go until I retire." He also doubted he could relocate.

As his doctor I feared Bart's decision might cost him much more, such as the loss of his life, or his ability to work or to enjoy any retirement in the future. The United States is a free country with people free to make the right or wrong decisions in their lives. But some people are trapped by our present system when the policies or plans are unfair or unjust, as in Bart's employer-based health insurance system.

And, where were the savings for our healthcare system when I hospitalized Bart six weeks later with a potentially preventable and now unstable heart condition? Bart's delay was a heart attack waiting to happen. Luckily he survived, but now he needed a more expensive and urgent heart catheterization.

A Don't Tell Policy

Medicare insurance is portable in this country and our society is mobile, especially the relatively healthy senior citizens. The southern states have warm weather in the winter and our community, in the center of wintry western New York, still offers cool and pleasant summers. Stanley had Medicare HMO coverage but knew that it was "not portable" if he lived outside his home area for over three months. As it was, Stanley developed an illness during his five-month stay in Florida and decided to seek care at a clinic. The temporary Floridian paid out-of-pocket. He explained, "I didn't want 'them' to know I was in Florida." Stanley feared using the HMO insurance might jeopardize his overall coverage, or possibly even demand a premature return to New York State for further care. Is "market-driven" healthcare supposed to create "big brother" anxiety? The industry public affairs program indicates otherwise.

The Same Old Story

Another patient, Fortney, came in a couple of weeks before Stanley but with a different twist. He had severe multiple medical problems in the past, but now those conditions were stable with numerous medications, including expensive immunosuppressive drugs. Fortney was living in Florida for four months each year, knowing the HMO coverage would not continue past three months. He developed a painful rash but thought it was only "bug bites." He failed to see a physician in Florida with the same excuse, "I didn't want them to know." After all, he was out of the area over three months and broke HMO rules.

Who says we are free to travel even in our own country?

"Why not just stay with Medicare?" I asked him when he came in to show me the rash.

"I need the prescription coverage with the HMO. My medications are too expensive.

The HMO covers $2,500 per year of my medications," he explained.

When I looked at the rash, I saw Fortney had shingles, not bug bites. Thankfully, this temporary Floridian had no major problems, but I anticipate they will occur in the future. It is just a matter of time. I saw a study which showed that seniors will change insurance companies to meet their medication needs.[1] If they have high prescription costs, "the sick" will migrate towards the plans with better drug coverage. Is this an advantage of the market-driven system or will those insurance companies become less profitable and then drop coverage or benefits for their patients? Many insurance companies are already dropping HMOs or prescription coverage to remain profitable.

A Vacation Cut Short

A patient of mine, Philip, was on vacation about 700 miles away when he developed severe abdominal pain and a high fever. He went to the local emergency room and was immediately hospitalized. He was treated with intravenous antibiotics and the doctors recommended immediate surgery to remove an infection. They told him the illness was critical.

Rather than have the surgery, Philip decided to charter a plane and fly back home. This cost him $2,000 and risked his life. When one of our local surgeons told me what happened, I said, "I bet his insurance had something to do with his decision." (The surgeon hadn't thought of that possibility.)

"Why did you fly back home for surgery instead of staying out there?" I asked him in the hospital.

I was flattered when Philip said, "I wanted to be back home where my doctors are."

"Did your health insurance have anything to do with your decision?"

He looked at me with surprise and answered, "Why yes, it did." When I asked him how much of his decision was related to health insurance, he estimated, "about 50%."

He had a Medicare HMO and feared the insurance would not cover this emergency surgery. Minus $2,000 and surgery delayed more than twenty-four hours later, Philip's ultimate outcome was fortunately successful. Nonetheless, he took a big risk because of uncertain insurance. Later the surgeon told me how difficult the operation was. He said, "The tissue was 'black' and it was 'just a matter of time' before it ruptured and filled the abdominal cavity with infection." If I told this story to Europeans, they would wonder about our sanity in not having universal healthcare.

More Delays and Fears

Debbie had employer-based health insurance and worked full time as a manager of a group home. She had sciatica, severe back pain radiating down her leg, which had been ongoing for over six months. Her surgeon and I recommended surgery, but she refused. When I asked her why she declined surgery, she bluntly explained, "I can't have my surgery. The surgeon says I would be off from work for two to six months. I would lose my job. Someone has to run the home." She added, "When the pain is severe, I'll just take my pain pills. I can't retire either. I need health insurance for me and my husband. The way his medical bills are, we won't make it on Social Security. I'd retire in a minute if I had health insurance. I only have thirty-four months to go until I have Medicare. My husband is sixty-one and all of his Social Security payments go for his medications and his medical bills. I'm trapped. You work all your life and look forward to retirement and it won't come. I gotta go to work to pay the bills and pills, but I don't know why I stay alive because of the pain." The surgery would alleviate the pain.

A Widower's Insurance Plan

Max, a widowed former patient, told me about his second wife who would not see a doctor. "She is paranoid," he explained. He then went on to tell me she did not have health insurance either. It was too expensive for her.
"Don't you have insurance and why isn't she on your plan?" I asked. He then told me how his insurance is really through his first wife, who had died over three years earlier. He could not afford insurance on his own, so he has continued on his first wife's plan.

"I'll stop when the insurance company finds out," he explained.

"At least stop the insurance when you have Medicare," I suggested. He declined because his first wife's insurance had better coverage than Medicare. Why do patients have to cheat or lie to get the healthcare they need in the U.S. Is this is a market-driven result?

Another Elderly Patient

"It isn't fair. I don't have EPIC, but I have friends who fudge their income to become eligible for EPIC," this senior with high prescription drug costs lamented. She added, "I'll try and hang in there until next year when I become eligible." She did not lie on her prior application form explaining, "I have to be able to sleep at night."

A *Cardiac Arrest Survivor*

Sometimes patients are "lucky" and survive what we call "sudden death" or cardiac arrest. That happened to my patient, Marge, nearly three years ago when everything went well in the emergency system. Credit goes to the bystanders who administered CPR, the paramedics who defibrillated the patient and transported her to the hospital, and to the emergency room doctors and nurses who cared for her after that. Marge even went on for more tests, a heart catheterization, more therapies, medications, surgery and an automatic implantable defibrillator. For three years since, she has not had any more cardiac events. Luckily she had EPIC, which covered her various expensive cardiac medications. One anti-arrhythmic drug costs over $200 per month.

I saw Marge recently on a routine exam when she commented, "I went without my medications for a whole week. They cancelled my EPIC."

"Why?"

"I moved and did not receive my monthly bill from EPIC. When I needed more medications, I went to the pharmacy, but they would not give me the prescriptions unless I paid full price. I couldn't afford them. It took me one week before my EPIC was reinstated. My daughter had to call the state and I had to send in $20." The bureaucracy in this instance placed Marge's life at extreme risk for $20.

Marge later told me how her brother, who had died years earlier, had not paid this same pharmacy. The brother had cancer and multiple medical problems. At the time of his death there were over $700 in unpaid prescription drug charges. The pharmacy was now asking for payment from Marge. In other industrialized nations, this does not occur.

A *Retired Husband*

I diagnosed Earl, a family man, with a curable cancer and high blood pressure many years earlier. I had not seen him for over one year because his insurance had changed when his wife retired, and I did not participate with her retirement health insurance plan. Earl, however, did not want to pay $220 per month for health insurance premiums if he was unable to see his own doctor. So he went without health insurance and sometimes medications during this time.

When he turned sixty-five, he joined a Medicare HMO that I belonged to and he actually saw me, his doctor. Seven months later he traveled to

Florida, but his HMO was not portable. So after three months in Florida he again was uninsured. Two months later, he died of a probable sudden heart attack. God only knows whether he was still on his medications or not. The profit-oriented health system required, in this case, that he not stay in Florida. Where is the purported freedom in a system that limits a patient's ability to relocate at will? In reality the insurance companies make the decisions for the individuals. One may question why Earl would select a restrictive HMO, but he probably needed their prescription benefits.

A Choice Consumer Without a Choice

Don had a prior malignancy, which was treated by his specialist for years. He was on Medicare in which most patients have the choice of their physician. However, he changed to a Medicare HMO, ironically containing the word "choice" in its name. Don had to change his doctors and came to me as his new primary care physician. He also had to find a new specialist physician. When Don needed to see another specialist, I could only refer him to one who participates in the HMO.

By changing from Medicare to the Medicare HMO, Don actually had "less choice" but also "less costs." For Medicare, however, I am not sure they realized less costs overall. The new specialist would probably order more tests and charge an initial higher level of service compared to the patient's previous doctors. The right thing for Don was to continue with his same physicians from the beginning. In the market-driven system, choice of doctors in America can be limited and this is happening more and more.

A Matter of Timing

Anita had a problem that her primary physician could not solve and was referred to a specialist. Weeks before seeing the specialist, however, Anita's insurance was changed to an HMO in which neither the primary nor the specialist physician participated. Similar to Don's situation, Anita had to change two doctors now, a new primary one and a different specialist. Records were recopied and more phone calls made. This was obviously a waste of time for the patient and physicians and probably for the HMO as well.

The Same Dilemma

Kay retired at age sixty-two and no longer was insured through her former employer. Thankfully, she could obtain coverage under her husband's employer-based insurance plan. Only one health insurance plan was offered to him however, and I did not participate in that plan. This is a common problem for many workers in America. Forty-two percent of workers with employer-based insurance are offered only one insurance plan for their family or themselves.[2] Then, too, employers sometimes change plans, which restricts or changes the patients' choices even further.

Kay had to change primary care physicians when she retired. The new doctor had an office thirty miles from where she lived. She wrote me a letter apologizing for the change, but asked if she could come back to me in three years when she turns sixty-five and has Medicare. What is the beneficial effect of the market-driven system in this case? There is none. It is a complication. This patient would have more freedom and peace of mind in three years with automatic universal coverage and Medicare. Why does she have to wait?

December 12, 1999

Jamestown, NY 14701

Attn: Dr. Rudolph J. Mueller

Dear Dr. Mueller:

Please accept this letter as my authorization to have my medical records released and sent to

Fredonia, NY 14063-1804.

I deeply regret having to make a change at this time, but my coverage has changed to Choice ▆▆. Since you do not handle Choice ▆▆ patients, I have to make the change. When I am sixty-five, in three years, I would like the option of returning to you under ▆▆ Choice which I know you handle.

Again, thank you for taking me on as a patient and for all of your understanding and care. If I had any choice about what I wanted to do, I would not be leaving you as a patient.

Thank you for your assistance in handling this transfer to Dr. ▆▆ for me. Should you have any questions or need anything further from me, please call me at either ▆▆ or ▆▆

Sincerely,

Jamestown, NY 14701

PS: I have an appointment with Dr ▆▆ around the 4th of January next year so if this could be done prior to that, I would appreciate it very much.

Kay's letter stating her apologies for having to change her doctor

All physician-patient changes are not the fault of employers, HMOs or insurance companies. Recently a local medical group practice made the decision not to participate with a local HMO. I knew some of the patients had no other options for health insurance and were forced to change doctors. I knew some patients potentially could have been harmed by the group's decision. This is another result of the market-driven system.

Much of the American healthcare system places insurance company profits and physicians' incomes over patients' freedom of choice and continuity of care. In a recent survey of people who changed doctors, 74% did so because of their employer and insurance company changes.[3] A study has shown that Americans on average have shorter patient-doctor relationships compared to Canada, Australia or Great Britain.[4] A more rational healthcare system would have patients changing doctors less often and if so, for mostly patient-related reasons such as relocation from a community or dissatisfaction with a doctor's service. How much additional cost is added onto the system when patients change doctors so frequently? How much benefit of the patient-doctor relationship is lost?

Some people claim Medicare is "socialized medicine." It seems to me that everyone would have more freedom and peace of mind knowing they had automatic health insurance through Medicare at any age. According to a physician survey in 1999, 95.7% of the doctors accept some or all new Medicare patients. And total physician participation has also been increasing over time, up to 86.3% in 2000.[5] For millions of people, it is the American HMOs, insurance companies and some doctors who limit the patients' choice of their healthcare providers.

The current White House wisdom is to give the elderly "more choices" in health insurance plans and coverage. I believe many sick or elderly patients are afraid to change plans, because they are unsure of what actual differences exist between programs. They are confused over why such differences exist in the first place. In Western New York, there are eight different insurance companies offering eight different Medigap policies, along with at least three different HMOs, each with different plans. I counted at least seventy different choices Medicare patients can make with their Medigap policy, and patients can even change their options every month. The real choices patients need and deserve are the freedom to choose their own doctors, hospitals, therapists, or pharmacy, not for the HMO or insurance company to choose.

A Manager

A thirty-four year old manager, Jesse, had congenital health problems but had overcome amazing obstacles, except the lifelong lack of affordable health insurance. He worked full time for sixteen years, but now is disabled. The chronic illness has taken its toll and Jesse is unable to work forty hours per week. He still however, wants to work, but only part time. His employer only offers health insurance benefits to full-time employees. Jesse could not risk losing necessary health insurance. He was even willing to split the cost difference for part-time versus full-time employer-based health insurance, but the employer refused. Most of us depend on employer-based health insurance, but only 19% of part-time workers are offered health insurance benefits by their employers.[6]

Jesse understood the personal health and financial risks if uninsured. Unfortunately, this employer lost a valuable manager with sixteen years experience and society lost another gainfully employed worker to disability.

The Five-Minute Layoff

A patient, Carolyn, told me how her fifty-nine year old husband, Adam, had just been laid off his job of over twenty years. They gave him, along with hundreds of other employees, "five minutes notice." What concerned her even more was their potential loss of health insurance. Carolyn was insured by her husband's employer and relied on this vital coverage for her own health.

I thought she would easily qualify for disability, considering her multiple health problems, but then she proceeded to tell me her life story.

In her mid-twenties Carolyn was married with two children. Her first husband died unexpectedly, and she raised her children on Social Security benefits for two years. She fell in love again and remarried at the age of twenty-eight. She had more children and raised her new family. However, her health took a turn for the worse in the early 1980s when she sustained multiple serious problems. She had a heart attack and blood clot in an extremity requiring an amputation. Other medical problems seemed to "find her" from that moment forward. Knowing her chronic problems, I assumed she would have qualified for disability. It was obvious to me that she could not sustain work. Carolyn told me she tried to obtain disability at one time, but was told she did not qualify. She explained, "My husband worked and he made too much money."

Today Carolyn is medically stable on over ten different medications. I have been able to keep her out of the hospital for years and from any new serious health problems. What concerns Carolyn and Adam now is what will happen to her when she no longer has health insurance through Adam. She admitted, "I'm fearful how we will make it." I knew Adam would not be able to sustain COBRA payments for their continued insurance. He too will join the ranks of the uninsured. And will anyone hire this man at the age of fifty-nine? Presumably the layoff was market-driven, but some irresponsible employers also discharge older workers before they can earn retirement benefits. A market-driven healthcare system will not provide for them. Every other industrialized nation has a means of doing so and protecting workers from employer decisions.

A Common Worker

"I have good news! I am going to have my surgery," Tillie blurted out as I walked into the exam room.

"That's great. How long has it been since your surgeon said you needed surgery?"

"Two years. It was only after my lawyer got involved did 'they' agree to cover my surgery," she responded with a smile. The problem for Tillie was her two different insurance companies. Neither would authorize coverage for her orthopedic surgery. Neither company thought it was their financial responsibility, leaving Tillie in pain and unable to perform her normal manual labor duties for two years. They had to be threatened with legal action before they would agree to pay.

The market drive in this case is obviously not for the benefit of the patient. It made me feel sick knowing she remained in pain for over two years despite having more than one health insurance company. American health lobbyists and employer-based health insurance supporters would have us believe only patients in other countries, such as Canada and England, face long waiting lines. Two years is a long time to wait in line, plus the legal fees. When it comes to waiting lines, the American healthcare system can be the worst for some patients.

Double Insurance and Still More Waiting Lines

Dennis, a WWII survivor, had a history of colon polyps and other medical problems. His medications were too expensive for him with no prescription benefits through Medicare, so he decided to use the VA's "free prescription" benefit. The VA doctor ordered a colon test performed by the VA specialist. When an abnormality was found, the VA specialist recommended a repeat test in six weeks. Soon after the initial exam, Dennis changed to a Medicare HMO. He now asked me to refer him back to the VA specialist and I tried. The HMO did agree to cover the VA specialist, but only if seen in the next three months. As a result of all the confusion and paperwork, Dennis did not follow up with the VA specialist during that "magic" three-month period. When he showed up later than the authorized time period, the HMO declined payment for the VA specialist. When Dennis told me of the delays, I referred him to a new HMO covered specialist. The appointment took three months to obtain and the repeat test was now performed another three months later.

Twenty months after the first VA procedure, the colon abnormality required major surgery. I tried to reassure Dennis that he probably needed this surgery anyway because the first specialist could not remove the entire abnormality from the colon. At least, I hope that was the case. How much did the government save in taxpayer money by not providing this patient with affordable medications and doctors of the patient's first choice? The net cost was undoubtedly much greater.

Dennis was fortunate to survive the frontlines and battles in WWII, but he may not survive the waiting lines and insurance battles in the United States. Obviously uninsured patients face long waiting lines for medical care in the U.S., even longer than the insured.

One Sunday our church's adult education class had a panel discussion by church members entitled "The Golden Years—A Panel on Retirement." One panel leader recommended, "Don't let your job harm your health." She explained how her work consumed her life and she eventually ended up in the intensive care unit. Other members suggested people plan well in advance for their retirement. One retired member recommended people purchase long-term health insurance. I know patients with preexisting medical conditions who were denied long-term health insurance regardless of willingness to pay.

Another church member, a sixty-four year old employed library assistant, responded, "I'll probably die pushing books! I only hope I will live seven more months before I can become eligible for Medicare." After the Sunday adult education class, she told me how she had no health insurance. She could not even imagine long-term health insurance. She had multiple symptoms, but had not seen a doctor in ten years due to the high cost. I advised her to call my office for an appointment. I would not charge her and yet she still refused, "No, I'm not a beggar." I insisted. "I'll think about it," she said. I think she does not even consider retirement as a possibility in her life. And, she still has not called for an appointment!

Wife of a 4F

A patient told me about her troubles in obtaining Medicaid health insurance before 1994. She has had so many things happen to her before and after that period. She is thankful that she is on Medicaid now. Disabled from a heart attack, diabetes, and stroke, she would have died long ago, if not for Medicaid. Recently, I asked her why she was not on Medicare. Even though she was under age sixty-five, she had been disabled for well over two years. She explained Medicare qualifications for disability require a previous work history over a ten-year period. Then the best five of the work years is averaged to determine the benefits allowed under Medicare. That is how my patient understood her ineligibility for Medicare. She then went on to say, "I took care of my children at home for many years. I'm not ashamed of my children. Isn't it important to care for your children at home?" Once able and the children not at home, she worked five years as a healthcare aide. "Why can't they take my five years that I worked?" she asked. I didn't know the answer. It seems discriminating against women considering that mothers still do the majority of infant and child care in this country.

Then she told me about her husband, who was uninsured. He suffered from heart failure and arrhythmias to name just a few problems. He is frequently ill, and his bills have been sent to collection agencies by many providers in the past. He worked over ten years but was judged not disabled "by a panel of non-physicians." His wife said, "He's sixty-three going on ninety-five."

"What about the VA? Did he serve?" I questioned

She then replied, "He wanted to serve in the military, but was rejected three different times and was classified 4F. He became deaf after a mastoid infection and coma when he was three years old," she said. Recently he called for an eye doctor appointment and was given one six months later.

According to the healthcare industry and their lobbies, Americans don't face waiting lines like patients in other countries with universal health insurance.

Husband and a Father

Millions of Americans are trapped in their lives by a dysfunctional and unjust healthcare system. Sometimes I feel like screaming, "Is anyone out there listening to the patients?" The more I ask patients questions about their healthcare coverage and life stories, the harder it seems to comprehend. Is this the America we really want for our children and our families?

This patient had been hospitalized for some time now with a chronic diabetic condition slowly worsening with time. The patient required frequent personal care for such basic needs we all seem to take for granted. These included assistance with bathing, dressing, transferring from bed to chair, and preparing meals. The patient also required frequent blood sugar monitoring, medication adjustments and administration. When I called the patient's family about future hospital discharge plans, the spouse responded, "I have to find care for my disabled child first. Then I can bring her home."

He went on to explain how he wanted to retire now and care for his family, but could not. His continued employment provided employer-based health insurance coverage for his entire family. He could not risk going without health insurance since their medical needs were so great. He was not worried about himself even though he was only a few years short of Medicare himself.

Eventually he found care for his child, continued to work and delayed his retirement. Soon afterwards, he brought his wife home. A few weeks later, she died unexpectedly.

Who says doctors should not cry?

A *Poor* Widow

I asked Patsy, a senior citizen patient, for a list of her medications because I needed to review the names, doses, and the frequency of her medication use. She had high blood pressure, diabetes, high cholesterol, and a prior stroke. She handed me this list.

Imdur	Oval pink – before breakfast	$36.83
Diabeta	Blue – ten min. after breakfast	$11.63
Lipitor	Small white oval – $1/2$ hr. after breakfast	$53.88
Lanoxin	Small yellow – after lunch	$5.29
Lasix	Round white – mid afternoon	$4.94
Plavix	Round pink – after dinner	$76.39
		$188.96 a month

She then commented, "I'm on EPIC now since my husband died. I'm a poor widow." I was not prepared for her list or her reply.

Three months later, Patsy returned for another diabetic office visit. I talked to her about EPIC and her medication costs. She said, "They wouldn't give it to me when Arnold was here. We missed by $30 per month. I write a list before I purchase the drugs. I had to make sure I had enough money before I went to the drugstore. I never pick up my prescriptions without checking my wallet first."

She then went on to tell me how she volunteers at the hospital rehabilitation center. One day she spoke to a man who had diabetes and had one leg amputated. This man, pointing to his amputation site, told her his illness cost three times more than his house. She also told me about an elderly lady standing outside of a drugstore without enough money. Apparently this elderly lady was four dollars shy of the necessary amount for her medications. Patsy felt sorry for her and gave the lady the four dollars. A few days later, this same lady returned the money. Among us there are magnificent people at all levels of society.

Months later, Patsy again came into my office. This time she told me she found a hidden shoebox at home with $896. It was her late husband's shoebox. "Poor Arnold, God bless him. He was so worried I wouldn't be able to make it once he was gone," she explained.

No Time to Slow Down

Frank, a sixty-nine year old man, had a full-time job but no employer-based health insurance benefits. He had Medicare, but no prescription coverage. I was treating him for high blood pressure, chronic emphysema, and osteoporosis. I prescribed some breathing medications, but he would not use them as prescribed because they "cost too much." I also offered treatment for his osteoporosis, but he declined. He explained how his wife also had multiple medical problems and multiple medications for which he was currently paying over $300 per month.

"There's not much left after I put gas in the car," he said. He joked, "When my wife dies, I can slow down. I won't need to work so hard to pay for her medications."

A Not Retired Husband

An eighty-two year old patient wanted to cut back on her medications because they were too expensive. She had prior heart surgery and high blood pressure. She told me, "It's a good thing my husband is still working! He's only eighty-four."

The Pill Cutter

Dick, a seventy-year old patient on Medicare, had significant coronary artery disease and reflux esophagitis, both problems that can easily cause recurrent chest pain. I had him on multiple medications; some were too expensive for him to purchase. Since he had no prescription coverage, he found clever ways to afford his medication. Some patients will cut their pills in half to save money. One of Dick's medications cost nearly $5 per pill. He decided to cut the pill in five pieces. He tried six pieces once but he told me he couldn't break them that small.

In the 2000 election, both major presidential candidates fortunately agreed Medicare patients need affordable medications. Unfortunately, neither plan fully met the needs of my patients. Both plans were voluntary and still placed potential and real significant costs on the elderly population.

"To Be?"

I never thought I would write a book, but the sad and sick healthcare stories that needed to be told kept coming into my office and my life. I believe most doctors miss facts about their patients' lives. America's dysfunctional health system mocks individual liberties and freedom.

I started keeping track of the stories in August, 1999. A few months later, Harry and Louise came into my office and told me theirs. They were in love and wanted to get married, but didn't. They feared their marriage would lead to Harry's loss of Medicaid coverage, with resultant loss of prescription coverage. Harry had already spent his life savings of $35,000 over the previous decade on his out-of-pocket medical expenses. He now was impoverished from years of inadequate health insurance and decades of multiple chronic medical problems including juvenile onset diabetes. His life was dependent on vital medications that cost well over $400 per month. Harry and Louise knew their marriage would place Harry's life at risk. Our nation's lack of guaranteed health insurance for all people forces many to make such sad life decisions. And, I know Louise has saved Medicare and Medicaid numerous additional medical expenditures by her great care and love for Harry. He would have had many hospitalizations and emergency room visits without her daily management of his insulin and blood sugars. This is not "job-lock" but "single-lock." No nation in the world does this to its citizens except the United States.

"Or Not To Be?"

Another patient of mine, Lucy, lived and worked part time for a government institution in another state and needed major surgery costing $30,000. She fortunately had health insurance but it was under her husband's plan. Unfortunately Lucy, in addition to the surgery, also wanted a divorce. She had to decide whether to remain married temporarily and have the surgery with insurance coverage or file for divorce, and face having no health insurance and forego the operation. The choices Americans have to make between decent healthcare and other life issues because of the healthcare system would happen in no other industrialized democracy.

I have seen many other patients make major life decisions unrelated to their health, but definitely related to their health insurance status. Another just blurted out one day; "I'd retire in two months if only I knew how to pay for my health insurance."

Scared to Make a Move

Steve and his wife Edie are both on Medicare. They pay $331 per month for their secondary insurance coverage. This plan had a $400 per person deductible and a $15 per prescription co-pay. Steve has severe chronic lung disease and his wife has severe osteoporosis. I spoke with them about possibly trying a local Medicare HMO in an effort to save them some medical costs.

Steve responded, "We're scared to make a move at the wrong time. My wife is in such bad shape."

This is another example of many sick elderly patients who are afraid to change plans, unsure of what actual differences exist between plans and confused over why such differences exist in the first place. The market-driven system draws its full share of charlatans. People are deceived and cheated. This creates a fear of the system among the most vulnerable.

George the Former Carpenter

George, the former carpenter from Chapter One, faced permanent poverty from his multiple medical illnesses and his inability to work. The government had granted him Medicaid coverage permanently, nearly four and one-half years after I first met him. Unfortunately, his diabetes and other health problems continued to advance. He had trouble breathing, high potassium and worsening kidney function. Over the next year, George required eight hospitalizations for a total of forty-one days to treat the various chronic medical problems. He had heart failure, kidney failure, strokes, neuropathy and nearly total vision loss. Soon we started dialysis to try to control his fluid and electrolyte problems.

Luckily, patients on dialysis automatically qualify for Medicare insurance, a quirk in the law. This begs the question; are patients with chronic renal failure more special than patients with other types of chronic expensive conditions? Why are patients with renal failure treated differently and receive guaranteed Medicare? Did someone in the family of a former congressman have chronic renal failure? Anyway, with Medicare, George's hospital and doctors would enjoy even better reimbursement.

If only George could have enjoyed any remaining health. This previously hard-working carpenter who suffered from many major chronic disabilities, faced another disability—depression. I tried antidepressants with only partial success. He really missed his carpentry work and never really wanted to depend on others for his health or daily needs. He lost his pride as a result of this tragic illness. He could not work to sustain himself. He could not even walk without assistance. He needed help changing his urostomy bag on his abdomen for his vision had also failed. We tried to joke about his predicament, but we both knew it wasn't funny.

His sister and I eventually placed George in a nursing home covered by Medicaid. Since he was Medicaid and not "private pay," he had to share a small room with three total strangers, each with their own medical problems. Private-paying nursing home patients get the "nice rooms" with privacy, space and nice views out the window. Have you ever seen what some other nursing home patients face? Sometimes the differences would depress anyone.

With multiple debilitating illnesses and his memory failing, George's will to live ceased. The now fully insured carpenter declined further treatment and died five months after nursing home placement and just months before his sixty-fifth birthday, the age of automatic Medicare eligibility. His sister sent me a wonderful thank you letter for his care.

A Blind Diabetic Without Electricity

Diabetes and poor vision afflicted both members of this next couple. The wife was blind and on insulin shots. One day the couple asked for my assistance with the public utilities company. Apparently they had not been able to pay their electric bills and the company threatened to turn off the power to their apartment. The weather was hot that summer, frequently with temperatures over ninety degrees and high humidity. I called the company, but they would not change their financial decision. "The power is going off; diabetes is not an adequate medical reason to continue electric service," the company representative told me. She then went on and recommended, "The patient should place her insulin in a cooler with ice."

As of 1999, 16% of U.S. and 21% of New York State inhabitants had incomes under the federal poverty level, and another 19% of U.S. inhabitants and 18% of New Yorkers were low income, defined as having incomes less than twice the federal poverty level.[7] It is a sad commentary that people in the richest nation of the world have to make choices between life-saving medications, and food, or utilities.

A Wife with Memory Loss

Cynthia's husband, Ron, told me how difficult it was to afford her medications. One day he explained, "I go to the pharmacy and I get those two stupid medications for $172 per month. We just missed EPIC! It is so much money that you want to forget taking them. The hell with it." One of the medications was for treatment of his wife's dementia. I thought it was interesting he used the word "stupid" when he described the medications. He courageously cares for his wife. Between his care and the medications, she stays out of the nursing home. Which will cost society more, medications for the elderly or premature nursing home care? The market-driven healthcare concept does not provide an answer.

A World War II Veteran

During WWII, Zachary served on a battleship defending our country. He told me about his two recent surgeries. The first was covered partially under Medicare. Currently Medicare covers only 80% of physician charges after a deductible is met first, unless of course, the patient also has a large Medigap policy. Zachary, like many other Medicare patients, could not afford the doctors' charges. So one year later, he decided to try the VA hospital in Pittsburgh. He had to take the VA shuttle van with other veterans and travel three hours, but there were no large out-of-pocket expenses to pay.

"Why didn't you have your surgery locally?" I questioned.

He responded, "I can't afford it. Those *** are a bunch of thieves. I called Medicare and they told me not to pay them another dime. And then the *** threatened me when I didn't pay the remainder of the bill."

Does anyone realize how much anger is generated when sick patients receive medical bills that they cannot afford to pay? He was satisfied with his care, however, in the VA. He told me, "Life is good when you wake up on the right side of the grass."

Americans deserve, can afford, and should have comprehensive health insurance for 100% of the population! Do not let the health industry lobby convince you otherwise. These first few chapters describe the results, in human terms, of our sick, market-driven system. These real life stories are not rare instances. They are representative evidence of America's unacceptable performance in healthcare with resulting human tragedy and injustice.

The next chapters explore my experience with the powerful elements of market-driven healthcare.

4: THE PHARMACEUTICAL COMPANIES

"Only a life lived for others is worth living."

Albert Einstein

As the healthcare crisis develops, the various elements of the industry will begin to reassess their positions. The pharmaceutical companies should be heroic in the view of Americans. They have brought about a majority of the miracles in modern medicine. Among them are some of the world's most effective and productive corporations. They behave, however, as though they have lost their focus as an industry meant to serve the best interest of the patients. The pharmaceutical companies have allied themselves with organizations such as Citizens for Better Medicare, which opposed universal prescription coverage under Medicare. However, major newspapers, magazines, and journals, such as *Consumer Reports*, *The New York Times*, and *The Washington Post* have published editorials calling for universal healthcare.[1]

Media attention on the pharmaceutical manufacturers has focused the high cost of drugs in the United States compared to other countries including Canada. Reports have shown American patients travelling to Canada by bus to save 40 to 60% off the price of their prescriptions. A Medicare patient told me, "My prescription here costs $122 a month, but when I went to see some friends in Canada, it cost $75 there. And when you consider the exchange rate, it would be less than $50." It's obvious that Americans pay a great deal more for the same medications compared to other countries of the world. See Figure Four on the next page. In this case the savings were over 50%.

The pharmaceutical companies have countered with television advertisements showing patients being bussed from Canada to the United States for healthcare treatments. Additional television messages and print ads highlight the new medical advances in drug therapy. The veiled claim is that

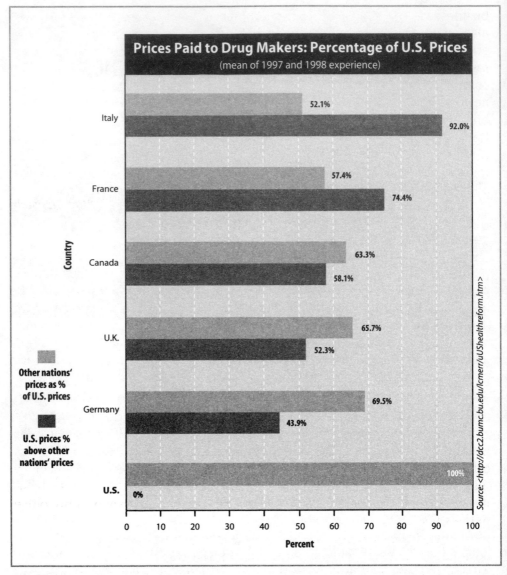

Figure Four

the institution of universal healthcare would damage the industry and impede progress.

Everyone should be pleased if every pharmaceutical company can make a reasonable profit from their research and manufacturing efforts. Society benefits from these scientific advances and the drug companies invest tremendous sums of money on research, over $26 billion in 1999.[2] This is an unusually high percentage of revenue, up to ten times that of other businesses. The United States government's National Institutes of Health also spent nearly $18 billion on medical research in 1998.[3] Many of the government funded research findings are passed onto the drug industry, or researchers collaborative with the pharmaceutical and medical equipment companies. These companies further develop new concepts and produce new medical therapies. These combined public and private research efforts bring new medications and treatment advances to the patients. The industry trade group, The Pharmaceutical Research and Manufacturers of America (PhRMA), claims in their website, "New medicines increasingly will replace more expensive and invasive medical treatments and thus will reduce overall healthcare costs."[4]

Unfortunately, overall healthcare costs are not falling. According to this same website, France, Germany, Great Britain, Sweden, Belgium, and Switzerland, with a combined population of nearly 230 million, accounted for 40% of all new drugs developed from 1975 to 1994, while the U.S., with a population of nearly 270 million, accounted for 45%.[5] Despite what the PhRMA trade group may claim, the other wealthy nations of the world can and do produce new medications under universal, national health programs and "price control," policies that set the prices pharmaceutical companies can charge.

When one considers the new medical advances and research in the world, it is the wealthy democratic nations that lead the world, irrespective of their healthcare systems. But what does the United States' pharmaceutical industry do? The issue is to evaluate whether Americans or patients want these practices in their healthcare system.

The pharmaceutical industry spends more time and money in the United States marketing their products to physicians and patients than any other country of the world. The U.S. pharmaceutical industry has extremely high marketing expenses, 22% of revenue; many times that of other businesses.[6] There are some excesses. Here are five that happened in my office in the same week:

First, I met a pharmaceutical representative who was promoting the advantages of one of her company's prescription drugs. "You can win $25,000. All you have to do is tell me one thing about my drug," the representative explained to me. I told her something about the medication and she handed me a lottery ticket. The ticket was a winner, although I never claimed the five dollar prize. Funny, I have never purchased a winning lottery ticket!

In a second visit, a representative from another company offered me $500 to attend an afternoon education conference sponsored by the company; $500 for my inconvenience to receive "training" in my field of medicine.

In the third instance, a drug company offered to send a free bouquet of flowers to my wife on Valentine's Day if I would spend a few minutes with their representative. I don't know any physicians who can't afford to send Valentine's Day flowers to their spouses, even though some may not remember.

The fourth incident came by mail. I received, along with 1,500 other physicians nationwide, an offer to participate in a clinical research study funded by a drug company. We were asked to prescribe their medication, if clinically indicated, to four of our patients. This prescription drug was already

Rudolph Mueller, MD

Jamestown, NY 14701

Dear Dr. Mueller,

▓▓▓▓▓▓ Pharmaceuticals invites you to participate in an Osteoporosis Clinical Learning Day to discuss diagnosis, management, and treatment of osteoporosis. Your background and expertise in the care of osteoporotic patients will be especially helpful, and your input will be valuable for the development of future educational programs.

This meeting is scheduled for Thursday, ▓▓▓▓▓▓, 2000 at the ▓▓▓▓▓▓▓▓ Conference Center in Buffalo.

You will be provided a consulting fee of $500.00 for your services. Your representative will contact you shortly to confirm your attendance at the program. A copy of the agenda and list of questions to be discussed during the feedback session is included for your review.

We look forward to your participation.

Sincerely,

Sales Consultant
▓▓▓▓▓▓Pharmaceuticals ▓▓▓▓

Attachments

Examples of drug companies' offers

tested and approved in this country and has been in use for many years. This "clinical research" by the company was attempting to test certain blood test changes when patients were on their medication. The patients' clinical and blood test outcomes would be followed over a six-month period. Each physician prescribing this chronic, long-term medication to their patients, would receive $2,000. Of course there were some forms to complete and the doctors could still charge the patients their routine fees for the required office visits. The patients would receive the blood tests and medications "free" for the first six months. I assumed that my patients would remain on this chronic medication for many years to come. Considering the current cost of this drug, easily over $100 per month, I thought the $500 per patient invested by the company would be easily recouped in two or three years. Was this necessary clinical research or some misguided marketing technique?

The fifth solicitation appeared on our fax machine, when a flier proclaimed, "Want to feel like a Superhero, Doctor Mueller?" This marketing company offered me a "free" office computer with video, e-mail and Internet access for one year. In exchange, I would have to talk over the video computer network with at least three drug representatives per month. "Only minutes" of my time, the flier stated. I think that just about any doctor in America would want a free computer, e-mail and Internet access. Of course, this offer is not "free." The patients or their insurance companies or HMOs are paying for the drug industry's high marketing costs.

I have many more examples of what I think are excessive and sometimes abusive techniques used by the industry to promote its medications to physicians. The marketing objectives are to make physicians aware of new drugs or new information about existing products. The practice of medicine should provide a feeling of scientific communication and intelligent conversation. Instead, we have a market-driven competition between similar medications with some foolish results.

One drug representative wrote me this note, "Could I see you for just nine seconds? If I go over that, I will take your staff to dinner." Another representative offered not only a bouquet of flowers but also drinks and hors d'oeuvres. Like most physicians, nurse practitioners, and physician assistants across the United States, I have been offered lunch or dinner meals, tickets to comedy shows, the theatre, professional sports events and amusement parks. Doctors are offered body massages, manicures, toys for their children, toys for themselves, tennis lessons, and weekend trips to Florida and other exotic places. I could go on with what seems to me like bribery by the pharmaceutical industry. In 1990, the AMA's Council on Ethical and Judicial Affairs published guidelines that limited gifts to doctors by the drug companies. The AMA's Working Group for the communication of ethical guidelines for gifts to physicians from industry have been revised as of

August 31, 2001 [(E-8.061) www.ama-assn.org/go/ethicalgifts] as follows:

1. Any gifts accepted by physicians individually should primarily
entail a benefit to patients and should not be of substantial value.
Accordingly, textbooks, modest meals, and other gifts are appropriate
if they serve a genuine educational function. Cash payments should
not be accepted. The use of drug samples for personal or family use is
permissible as long as these practices do not interfere with patient
access to drug samples. It would not be acceptable for non-retired
physicians to request free pharmaceuticals for personal use or use by
family members.

2. Individual gifts of minimal value are permissible as long as the
gifts are related to the physician's work (e.g., pens and notepads).

3. The Council on Ethical and Judicial Affairs defines a legitimate
"conference" or "meeting" as any activity, held at an appropriate location, where (a) the gathering is primarily dedicated, in both time and
effort, to promoting objective scientific and educational activities and
discourse (one or more educational presentation(s) should be the
highlight of the gathering), and (b) the main incentive for bringing
attendees together is to further their knowledge on the topic(s) being
presented. An appropriate disclosure of financial support or conflict
of interest should be made.

4. Subsidies to underwrite the costs of continuing medical education
conferences or professional meetings can contribute to the improvement of patient care and therefore are permissible. Since the giving of a
subsidy directly to a physician by a company's representative may create
a relationship that could influence the use of the company's products,
any subsidy should be accepted by the conference's sponsor who in turn
can use the money to reduce the conference's registration fee. Payments
to defray the costs of a conference should not be accepted directly from
the company by the physicians attending the conference.

5. Subsidies from industry should not be accepted directly or indirectly to pay for the costs of travel, lodging, or other personal
expenses of physicians attending conferences or meetings, nor should
subsidies be accepted to compensate for the physicians' time.
Subsidies for hospitality should not be accepted outside of modest
meals or social events held as a part of a conference or meeting. It is
appropriate for faculty at conferences or meetings to accept reasonable honoraria and to accept reimbursement for reasonable travel,
lodging, and meal expenses. It is also appropriate for consultants who

John [redacted]
Sales Representative

Dr. Mueller,

Could I see you for just 9 seconds. If I go over that, I will take your staff to dinner.

John [redacted]

Additional offers I have received from pharmaceutical companies.

Dr. Mueller   and a guest are cordially invited to attend

the Buffalo Sabres
vs.
the Florida Panthers

Join us on [redacted] 2000

Dr. [redacted]

will discuss

"[redacted]-A New Non-Systemic Approach to Lower LDL-C"
5pm-6:30pm Cocktails, Dinner, and Discussion

6:30pm Game

RSVP by [redacted] 2000 to
[redacted]

First Come, First Serve
Space is Limited

provide genuine services to receive reasonable compensation and to accept reimbursement for reasonable travel, lodging, and meal expenses. Token consulting or advisory arrangements cannot be used to justify the compensation of physicians for their time or their travel, lodging, and other out-of-pocket expenses.

6. Scholarship or other special funds to permit medical students, residents, and fellows to attend carefully selected educational conferences may be permissible as long as the selection of students, residents, or fellows who will receive the funds is made by the academic or training institution. Carefully selected educational conferences are generally defined as the major educational, scientific or policy-making meetings of national, regional or specialty medical associations.

7. No gifts should be accepted if there are strings attached. For example, physicians should not accept gifts if they are given in relation to the physician's prescribing practices. In addition, when companies underwrite medical conferences or lectures other than their own, responsibility for and control over the selection of content, faculty, educational methods, and materials should belong to the organizers of the conferences or lectures.

The PhRMA had pledged to follow these guidelines in the past.[7] Currently the pharmaceutical companies have over 58,000 drug representatives and spend $8,000–13,000 per physician per year marketing their products.[8] Drug promotion to physicians by the drug industry costs well over $10 billion per year in the United States, and exceeds the total dollars spent on educating all of the medical students and doctors-in-training in this country.[9]

Are these dollars well spent when it comes to educating physicians? One medical study found that drug-company sponsored continuing medical education for physicians led to worse physician prescribing practices. These enormous efforts from the pharmaceutical companies are all in the name of "education" for the physician, nurse practitioner and physician's assistant, but are frequently biased toward their particular company's product, and they do influence the practitioner's prescribing habits.[10]

On a recent Tuesday afternoon, I met with a pharmaceutical company representative in my office. Two years earlier, this same company offered to fly my wife and me to Boston, with weekend accommodations at an exclusive hotel, all expenses paid and $400 extra spending money. In return, my wife and I were to attend an educational conference promoting their medication. This conference claimed this new therapy was a breakthrough in treatment for a common chronic medical disorder. However, since that Boston "conference" two years ago, there have been some serious liver problems associated with this medication and recent concerns in the medical literature.

At this Tuesday meeting, the drug representative asked, "Doctor, what do I have to do to get you to prescribe my medication?" I then went on and told her my concerns about recent liver problems and that I would not write any new prescriptions for this medication until the issue was cleared up. She then told me how the Federal Drug Administration (FDA) had just met with the company and found the medication safe. She pressed on further but I still said no. That very next morning the local news reported that the drug had been pulled off the market by the FDA because of reported liver toxicity and reported patient deaths. I don't think drug representative was purposely being dishonest with me, perhaps she was just uninformed.

Two days later, another drug representative appeared to promote a competitor's drug, similar to the one just removed from the market. She told me how safe their drug was, and that patients can be switched to this medication. She also mentioned being in Texas the day before and scheduled for a solid week of training sessions. She was, however, flown back immediately to her sales territory with the news of the FDA's action against her competitor. "Forget the training and get to the sales opportunities," I thought.

It is profit-motivated competition that puts the representatives back in the field when their competitors take a hit. I understand and appreciate competition and the incentives it delivers, but I include this story to illustrate the marketing tactics and strategies of present pharmaceutical company competition.

Not to be outdone, another competitor drug company representative was in my office soon after the FDA action. He also claimed that his drug in the same drug class was safe and that recent liver toxicity reports published in a peer reviewed medical journal, "Just aren't true." This drug representative explained, "They were poor studies." However, there was a further development. Just prior to the printing of this book, I received a letter from his company's president conveying this drug warning:

> "...reports of hepatitis and hepatic enzyme elevations three or more times the upper limits of normal rate have been received."

One medical study found that 11% of drug representatives' factual claims were actually false and only one quarter of the physicians who heard the claims actually recognized the false information.[11] Does the $8-$13,000 spent on each physician also serve to create confusion? There are better ways to inform active physicians about current and new therapies. What does it mean when practicing physicians are "trained" by drug representatives who benefit financially from the sales of their medications? Does this lead to quality, affordable medications for all Americans? It doesn't seem to.

And how do the patients, those with little or no medical training and education, assess appropriate drug indications and benefits? Since 1997, the pharmaceutical companies have been able to market their prescription medications to the patients or, as some refer to it, "direct-to-consumer." This occurred after much lobbying by the industry in Washington and was supported by the media who is always interested in new advertising dollars. The United States is the *only* country in the world that allows this type of advertising.

Even those who use television only as a news source and an occasional cultural or entertainment program can see how prevalent these advertisements have become. One can also find this advertising in newspapers and magazines. Direct-to-consumer advertisement costs exceeded two billion dollars in the year 2000.[12] Patients have trouble affording their medications, but the drug companies seem to have no trouble affording the advertising costs.

No doubt these new marketing techniques are effective or this money would not be spent on them. But are they safe? Annual prescription drug sales have climbed at least 12% per year since the approval of direct-to-consumer advertising in 1997, a rate of inflation essentially unseen prior this.[13] Patients do come to their doctors asking for the latest advertised drug. I wonder if it is because the actors always seem to be smiling with so much

relief from their maladies? One night watching one of television's most popular shows, I counted five different drug company advertisements solving
such medical problems as arthritis, erectile dysfunction, obesity, allergies
and esophagitis. At least the advertisers were not competing against each
other.

A 1997 survey demonstrated that "Four-fifths of family physicians in the
U.S. felt direct-to-consumer advertising was 'not a good idea' because these
techniques increased medication costs while also promoting misleading and
biased drug information."[14] Another study showed that up to one half of all
patients would be disappointed if their physician did not prescribe the
advertised medication and 15% would consider changing doctors altogether.[15]

The pharmaceutical companies should deliver public educational messages on the prevention of health problems such as heart disease, cancer,
high blood pressure, diabetes, obesity, alcoholism, and drug abuse. They can
relate this to their products by asking the public to be aware of the diseases
and their symptoms. The difference from what they are doing now is subtle,
but the results would be constructive.

We need to continually improve our efforts in all areas of care. There is
one possible step, which should be a new area of debate: should new technologies or medications be tested against current or standard treatments?
Presently, the FDA will approve new drugs or treatments if they are shown to
be safe and effective against placebos. The question is whether or not new
therapies should be shown to be better and safer or if they are equal, then
significantly less expensive, compared to current therapies. If not better,
safer, or significantly less expensive, then should these new technologies or
medications be approved at all? The National Institute of Health, private
industry or both could fund these medical studies to make the determination.

Others have called for such research. Uwe Reinhardt, a respected
authority in the public health field, suggested the government and pharmaceutical industry endow a private, non-profit research institute with 1% of
collective yearly drug revenues. This independent source's research would
help determine whether new and or improved medications are actually clinically and significantly better than current therapies. This research could also
lead towards "reference pricing," which has been used successfully in some
countries to control drug costs.[16]

A conversation is needed as to how to fully evaluate medical therapies
and treatments before incorporating these treatments into everyday medical
care, that affects the lives and health of patients. In 1997, thirty-nine new
medications were approved in the U.S. by the FDA. However, five of these
same medications, more than one out of every eight, have been withdrawn
in the U.S. or in other countries because of safety concerns. The average

duration or marketing of the withdrawn drugs has been eighteen months.[17]

Currently, the FDA approves all new prescription medications or medical devices in the U.S. There are well over one hundred different medications for the treatment of high blood pressure. How often do human errors occur because of the abundance of "me too" drugs, medications with similar clinical efficacy and chemical structures, but different brand names and dosages? And new brand name drugs are frequently two to three times the price when compared to older drugs with similar efficacy. Years later the brand name drugs seem to have lost their "profit" potential when generic equivalents are possible.

Probably the largest class of "me-too" drugs is the blood pressure medications classified as ACE (angiotensin converting enzyme) inhibitors. I know of thirteen different ACE inhibitors currently available in the U.S. Mistakes can and do happen with "me-too" drugs. One elderly patient I know was stable on her ACE, but her insurance company in an effort to cut their costs asked for a change to a different ACE. The change was made, but the patient couldn't tolerate the new medication, probably because of a non-equivalent dosage. Her blood pressure dropped too low; she became dizzy and fell, fracturing her shoulder. Fortunately, worse injuries were not sustained.

The insurance company lost considerably in this incident and the patient suffered. Make no mistake about the efforts to "save money." Unintentional injuries commonly occur because cost and money priorities outweigh the care of the patient. Do we really need thirteen different ACE medications when they have similar efficacy? The chance for human error increases dramatically with each new equivalent medication approved, each with a different name, frequency and dosage. When Americans, whether doctors, patients, insurance companies, hospitals or others place financial decisions before individual clinical decisions, then quality fails. Further, standard therapies will stop the jockeying by HMOs or insurance companies for savings. They should be the best and most cost effective for any condition.

A more effective way to lower the overall costs of individual brand name drugs is to allow for generics to reach the market in a more timely manner. New competitive drugs rarely bring significant overall cost reductions in these classes of medications. However, generics can make a big difference in price. But the drug industry lobby will oppose any attempts to increase the availability of competitive generic drugs to the patient. Obviously doctors and patients want generic medications to be of equal quality.

Another tactic used by drug companies to attract patients, regardless of what impact it could have on them, is direct-to-consumer mailings. An elderly patient with mild dementia asked me to complete a survey she had received in the mail. She didn't understand why the survey was sent to her or why someone was asking about her medical problems. I looked the survey over and called her. I discussed what I thought it was, but she still asked me to complete it. The form essentially requested information about any chronic medical disorder from which she suffered, as well as her address. I am sure she is now on multiple drug companies' direct-to-consumer mailing lists and is receiving information on current therapies for her medical problems.

The pharmaceutical industry was the most profitable in America in 1999 with an average 18.6% profit after taxes on revenue. It outpaced the technology companies and other major industries.[18] Pharmaceutical companies pay taxes of 16.2%, less than the overall taxes paid by other *Fortune* 500 companies, which were 27.3%.[19]

Recently, a colleague told me that he agreed with my viewpoints on most healthcare issues, but he could not see new medications being developed in this country "unless the companies can make a profit." He also said that most of the new technologies and medications are coming from this country. I was not so sure of his facts except I knew most of the AIDS drugs came from American research.

Searching for an answer, I telephoned an old friend with whom I had trained with in internal medicine at Northwestern University and who now works for the FDA. "Where are the new medications in the world being developed, the United States or elsewhere?" I asked.

He responded, "The pharmaceutical companies are now huge international companies. The medications are developed all across the world."

"But are the companies making a profit outside the United States?" I questioned further.

"Oh, yes. But the United States is where you want to sell your medications. This is where the big profits are!" he laughed. Market-driven medicine at its best, I thought.

The reason for such a favorable climate for pharmaceutical sales in the U.S. is that there are no controls on the price charged in the absence of a national healthcare policy. Medications cost much more in the United States than in the rest of the world, and are the leading factor of rising medical inflation rates. Prescription drug expenditures in the United States rose 18.6% in 1999, and at this rate could soon surpass spending on physician services.[20] Prescription drugs accounted for 44% of the total increase in healthcare costs in this country in 1999, with about one-third of the increase in drug spending attributable to higher prices and the balance to a higher volume of sales.

Americans often hear that the pharmaceutical industry is one of the last true "free markets" in American medicine. We hear that through competition more products will be delivered at affordable prices to the "customers" or patients. Economists, on the contrary, will say there are few "free" markets, especially in healthcare. Pharmaceuticals are not commodities; the competition is imperfect. Only a few producers offer therapies for particular diseases. They compete, but as in the steel or plastics industry, there are price leaders. Pharmaceutical companies, other than those producing generics, rarely use price to compete, which is one reason for the high marketing expenses.

Some companies resort to illegal practices in order to ensure that their profits are not harmed. In an embarrassing and expensive incident, federal authorities accused one company of paying a generic drug company not to make a generic equivalent to one of its products. The company's big selling medication was soon to go generic and thus face competition. The company paid $40 million and got caught. Another company falsified the results of equivalency tests between their brand and the similar generic medication. They also faced a large fine and embarrassment.

Pharmaceutical companies can also block generics through patenting techniques, which are legal. The brand-making drug companies bring their same medication out in different forms or for different indications, thus extending the length of their patent up to twelve more years. Someone named this trade practice as "ever green."

A recent study found that generic drugs could lead to lower prices for medications, in some cases up to 90% lower.[21] More generic medications would seemingly benefit a lot of sick people who can't afford their medications. This same report also stated that over time generic medications are becoming used less frequently. Currently, drug companies have seventeen years of patent protection from the original FDA application date of their medication and the potential monopoly on the particular drug's sales.

Often there are news reports about new treatments and therapies on radio and television, newspapers and news magazines. A study found that news coverage of new medications is frequently inadequate or incomplete concerning the risks, benefits, or costs. The study also uncovered the conflicts of interest between those people interviewed for the press stories and the drug companies sponsoring the research. Of these reports, 40% failed to report the benefits quantitatively, 53% failed to mention potential adverse reactions and 70% failed to mention costs. Half of all the experts in the studies mentioned had financial ties to the drug manufacturer.[22] Another recent study showed that in 1999, nearly 8% of all faculty investigators reported personal financial ties with the sponsors of their research. This included paid speaking engagements, consulting agreements, and advisory or board positions with the companies.[23]

Earlier in this chapter, I described the "clinical research" study opportunity I was offered. Doctors across America were solicited with compensation of $2,000 to recruit four patients with a specific medical problem, prescribe a specific medication, and draw blood on these same patients over a six-month period. I declined to participate. This study was conducted, and was later published in a well-respected medical journal. It did show a significant 16.9% reduction in the blood levels of a blood marker when patients were treated with the drug company's medication. I laughed when I saw only two out of every three patients in the study actually had their blood results collected by the end of the study. The authors failed to mention in the article that each participating doctor was paid the $2,000. In the small font print at the end of the article, I read "This study could not have been conducted without the dedication and commitment of the ...Investigators," (all 1,143 of them who were handsomely paid).[24]

I also read in other small print, the study supervisor and lead author had "pending patents" filed with a university hospital on similar blood markers. An editorial in this same journal questioned the clinical significance of the blood markers and patient outcomes since the study did not measure any differences in patient outcomes. In my opinion everyone in this study, except the patients who required this medication long-term, did well financially, including the drug company, the researcher, the university and the participating doctors. I doubt the participating doctors stopped the medication after the completion of the study. This medication can cost over $150 per month in our community.

Some may ask why I see pharmaceutical representatives in my office. The main reason is that I need the samples to give my uninsured and underinsured patients. I also use small amounts of the samples on first-time users to assess their tolerance. Patients should not have to buy a one-month supply of a medication if they can't tolerate it after a few days. That would be a waste of valuable medications and healthcare dollars.

To counter accusations that uninsured Americans cannot obtain necessary medications, the drug companies promote their "patient assistance programs." One drug representative told me how her company offered a "patient's saving program" involving prescription coupons for patients. The company had an expensive cholesterol-lowering medication that costs over $100 per month, and had been on the market for over ten years. Many of my patients cannot afford this. The coupon was for "$30 off" the drug cost per month. I read the coupon's "fine print" and realized patients would qualify only if they had no prescription insurance coverage and paid 100% of the drug cost initially. The coupon stated, "Enclosed is something to help you gain the life-saving benefits of prescriptions." Interestingly, the drug representative only had a "few coupons" to share with me. This same drug is on formulary at the local VA and many of my veteran patients are currently taking it, and it is "life-saving."

Another sad case involved a patient, Joe, who had high blood pressure, severe heartburn, depression, and was on three medications. He was working full time, but was uninsured and frequently running out of his pills. Two days before his office visit, he was fired. He was extremely anxious with very high blood pressure. "I don't know how my wife and I will make it," he cried, "What will I do?" I gave him some of the "free samples" and referred him to Catholic Charities.

Later, I filled out three different forms for the drug companies' "patient assistance programs." If doctors and patients complete the forms and patients meet the low-income eligibility requirements (each different) then the drug companies will mail "free medications" for individual patients every three months to the doctor for the patient to pick up. It is working for Joe now, but I must remember to complete the forms every three months. Joe must justify his financial eligibility every three months, as well. And, the pharmaceutical industry is critical of government bureaucracy.

One time, I tried calling a drug company for some more forms for another patient. This patient assistance program by the pharmaceutical company was called (company name) "Cares." My patient had severe heart failure, diabetes and is disabled and is currently on Medicare. He does not have prescription coverage through Medicare and does not qualify for Medicaid. He had been without his heart medications for weeks. When I attempted to call the drug company through their patient assistance program, I heard an automatic recording, "Please leave your name and address and we will send you the form to complete for your patient." I was then transferred to this mailbox to leave the information only to hear the next message, "This mailbox is full. Please call again." Either there are a lot of patients in need of assistance or this was a way to limit access to the program. In 1999 the drug companies gave out $750 million (wholesale cost) or 1.9 million "free" medications through their patient assistance programs.[25] This amounts to less than 1% of their total products' revenue, hardly a significant "free" offer in the big picture.

I remember watching the National Bipartisan Commission on the Future of Medicare on television. One senator stated that prescriptions would be affordable for patients if doctors only took the time and advantage of the pharmaceutical companies' patient's assistance programs and prescribed the cheapest drugs possible (not the best) or generics. Then another senator chimed in and said, "That is the most intelligent thing that I've heard yet on this Commission." It seemed they were blaming the cost of drug coverage on physicians! It would be enlightening if these senators ever tried to call the companies or complete their forms. Members of Congress have comprehensive insurance with prescription coverage for themselves and their dependents, and never experience what my patients must deal with. I invite these senators or their staff to hang around my office for a few days.

But what would happen if the United States had universal prescription drug coverage for all patients? Many in the pharmaceutical industry would cry out, "No, it would lead to price controls, loss of research and no new therapies."

Yes, there would be price controls. There are in Europe, where the prices are negotiated. This has not put the pharmaceutical companies out of business. In fact, new drugs are being discovered there and throughout the world. The promise of pharmaceutical research continues and no government should discourage that research. What is needed with price controls is fairness and assurance to the companies that they will get a fair return. If they can maintain high profits while everyone has the affordable medications that they need, who could object? This is the policy the industry should follow. Governments should keep in mind the risks that the industry takes. They are considerably more than bringing out a new car or software package.

The waste in the drug industry's marketing costs, over 22% of total sales today, could be turned into more quality research and development or lower drug costs. The numerous perks and outlandish offerings to physicians can be eliminated and with universal care, "free samples" could substantially be reduced. In my office practice, we probably throw out 20% of our "free samples" because the medicines are not distributed prior to their expiration dates. Samples are a costly and inefficient way to distribute medications to sick patients. In Great Britain, the drug industry is limited to 9% of sales for marketing costs and patients somehow manage to receive medications, even the newer ones.[26] As an example, *Glucophage*, now an effective and popular diabetic medication in this country, was available in Great Britain long before it could be prescribed in the United States.

With universal drug coverage in the U.S., the quantity of drug prescriptions filled would rise significantly. I believe it would probably rise over 20%. Medicare patients without drug coverage, over one third of all Medicare patients, fill only two thirds of their prescriptions compared to Medicare drug-insured patients.[27] Also consider that the uninsured, one-seventh of all Americans, receive individually only 60% of the health services that benefit the insured.[28] Some studies have shown the uninsured are up to five times less likely to fill a prescription compared to the insured.[29] All doctors are aware of patients without drug insurance who are unable to afford their prescriptions.

The multinational industry does produce miraculous medications that have alleviated suffering, prevented disability and extended life. Many in the industry have dedicated their lives to high purposes. Like practitioners, they expect to be well compensated and not to have financial concerns that interfere with their concentration on their work. Some pharmaceutical companies are rated highly among America's corporations. Several are on the *Fortune* list: The 100 Best Companies to Work For. But, as in other industries, there are companies that are managed by essentially greedy executives who can run a business, but who only nominally pursue a mission statement with societal benefits included. It is the best companies which pursue creating value for the society, which are the most successful and which keep employees until retirement or afterward. Their people will say, "I love this company."

Somehow the pharmaceutical companies seem to lose sight of their customers. Perhaps over the array of doctors, hospitals, wholesalers and chain retailers, patients seem to be distant people who bring prescriptions into drug stores. The industry opposes any kind of universal single payment insurance. They oppose any action that might lead away from the market-driven system into price controls. The pharmaceutical industry lobbies heavily in Washington and state capitals. I suspect, however, that the most effective companies may recognize that the provision of universal care can increase their growth and still maintain healthy profits.

If all patients fill their prescriptions, there will be an obvious boost of sales for the drug companies. At the same time the industry could reach agreements with a single payer as is the case in many democratic nations worldwide. The government and industry would set the drug prices for new products at a fair return, taking into account the enormous risks and costs undertaken in their development.

Further, there could be an agreement to reduce marketing costs. A more professional and appropriate approach could be made to physicians and other providers. Healthcare providers are required to obtain continuing medical education (CME) throughout their professional career. In New York, physicians must demonstrate fifty hours per year of CME activity. Educational meetings of primary care doctors or doctors with particular specialties could be arranged to discuss new therapies or treatments with unbiased experts, forgoing the perks, "bribes" and other drug company inducements that so many physicians receive across America today. Samples, brand and generic, would be used for testing individual patient tolerance only, not as an emergency measure for uninsured or poor patients or as a "perk" for the families of the doctors and staff.

The top pharmaceutical companies are capable of long-range creative vision. They can work to find a new model that fits into a universal healthcare system that provides affordable medications for all Americans. This new model would be one in which they identify their interests with the patients first and cease the lobby and legislative pressure which, as I have pointed out, is frequently contrary to the patients' interests. "Only a life lived for others is worth living," said Albert Einstein. The American pharmaceutical industry can change and agree to policies that will benefit all U.S. patients who need their products, while also remaining highly profitable and successful entities. The pharmaceutical companies, or at least the leading ones, can make such a change occur in America.

However, the insurance companies and HMOs present more serious concerns.

5: THE HEALTH INSURANCE INDUSTRY AND THE HMOs

"You can always count on Americans to do the right thing, after they've tried everything else."

Winston Churchill

The United States is the most prosperous country in the world and also has the largest number of health insurance plans and insurance companies. Americans have Medicare, Medicaid, the Veterans Administration (VA), Child Health Plus, about 1,500 insurance companies and about 300 HMOs. No other nation does this to itself. Most have essentially one-payer systems, sometimes with several outlets. In the U.S., federal, state and local governments currently pay at least 51% of all healthcare services.[1]

Each private health insurance company and HMO has a CEO and administrative staff. The for-profit companies, that billed $137 billion of $375 billion in premiums in 1998, aim to make a profit. Insurance companies collect premiums on contracts and policies, which they theoretically offer competitively and pay claims. This multitude of corporations and plans, private and public, factors a massive overhead cost onto the system.[2]

Health Maintenance Organizations are corollary to the insurance companies. Originally, these not-for-profit organizations were doctor's groups formed in the 1940s to work with patients to provide regular care with a focus on prevention. The Life Extension Institute of New York was one of the first. Many others formed and often took on executives of corporations or other groups where there was a special value in keeping them well. Recently they were reformed to try to curtail healthcare cost inflation. The idea was that HMOs would oversee the doctors and the treatments while providing comprehensive services and preventive healthcare. No other nation has such institutions. In the American fashion, nearly two-thirds of all HMOs are now for-profit.[3] At the behest of the healthcare industry lobby, we have established cost containment with companies who have to produce profits. This has been a dramatic failure.

What is the essential mission of the health insurance industry and the HMOs in this frequently investor-owned healthcare system?

A Septic Patient

Amazingly this patient, Dena, was able to walk into my office. She was dizzy and complained of abdominal pain. She was obviously sick with a high fever, low blood pressure, abdominal tenderness, and confusion. I admitted her directly to the hospital with acute diverticulitis and sepsis. She recovered quickly on intravenous fluids, antibiotics and was discharged in two days. Later I received a letter from her insurance company stating, "We are pleased to authorize the hospitalization for two days for this patient." But the letter went on to say the company "required notification prior to hospitalization next time."

If a patient has alarming symptoms, what responsible insurance company would possibly ask for prior notification before treatment? The "market drive" is in the wrong direction. Sick patients must come first in a rational and moral society.

A Stroke Patient

In his late seventies, Conrad still worked full time. Even though he suffered from severe heart disease, it did not stop him from doing what he loved to do. He even had his own health insurance and wasn't reliant on Medicare. Sadly though, his illness caught up with him. He sustained a major stroke and was paralyzed completely on one side of his body. We treated Conrad in the hospital and later transferred him to a rehabilitation hospital. It was obvious that he would need prolonged physical and occupational therapy.

Later he was transferred to a nursing home for long-term care and further physical and occupational therapy. His chances of ever working again were slim in my mind. We hoped he would recover some function and be able to go back home. He understood his problem and was willing to put in the effort.

In less than two days after his transfer to the nursing home, I received a phone call from a for-profit insurance company nurse reviewer. The reviewer explained how their company could no longer cover my patient's care at the nursing home. She reasoned the patient could not perform two hours per day of therapy and thus he only met the definition of "custodial care." I explained that Conrad had not even had a reasonable time to recover from his stroke and still needed therapy. I didn't care if he could only participate in therapy one hour a day, at least he was still alive and making some slow progress. However, the number of hours mattered to the insurance company, for they were not responsible for the nursing home costs for patients defined as "custodial."

I pleaded my patient's case unsuccessfully to the insurance company's medical director too. "Sorry he could be at home," responded the medical director, a doctor who had not even seen the patient. How could this medical director come to the opposite conclusion as mine?

I knew "home" was impossible for this patient. His wife, Clarissa, also my patient, had her own health problems. She was physically and emotionally unable to care for her husband at home. I also objected to the medical director's comment because home care was not in the patient's best medical interest. He still needed aggressive therapy as well as other essential treatments. He had Medicare as insurance "back-up." Medicare covers nursing home care for up to 100 days for patients able to participate over "one-half hour" in therapy and demonstrate progress or small gains. With Medicare back-up coverage, he was not sent home. Sadly, he died in the nursing home three weeks after the first insurance company's denial. Both insurance plans were the lucky ones; there would be no more expensive rehabilitation or future hospitalization costs to worry about with Conrad.

But the story ends with this bizarre request I received concerning Conrad weeks after his death. Previously Conrad had travel plans and purchased travel insurance, but he was unable to take the trip due to his prior health problems. I had already completed forms explaining why Conrad could not travel. A travel insurance company asked me to send his medical records covering the three-month period prior to his major stroke. The insurance company needed more documentation and proof of his prior illness. My word and a death certificate seemed not to be adequate proof of his medical problems. The doings of the insurance bureaucracy inundate doctors with such absurdity.

Secure?

I still laugh when I think of Gordon and the name of his for-profit Medicare HMO, especially after I cared for him through this serious illness. The HMO had "secure" in its name but I'm not sure Gordon felt so secure after this experience.

Gordon normally lived in the western U.S., but vacationed for months in our community. He developed an unstable medical condition with chest pains and an abnormal electrocardiogram. I saw him in my office and scheduled an urgent heart catheterization at the local hospital. The specialists found a serious problem and advised emergency heart surgery. The patient wanted the procedure performed immediately but then the for-profit insurance company intervened. They insisted the patient return home on a jet plane and have surgery at their "Center of Excellence." Luckily, Gordon survived the travel, the delayed surgery and recovered uneventfully.

It had been nearly two summers later when Gordon returned to my office with different chest pains and still the same insurance company. Not surprisingly, his prescription coverage now cost significantly more along with higher insurance premiums. This time I determined his chest pains were non-cardiac and provided treatment and advice. Some of the tests he declined since he wasn't returning to his home until the end of the fall. As you have read, some HMOs forbid patients continued coverage under their plan if the patient remains out of the area for over three months. Gordon was aware of the rules but didn't change his coverage.

Hopefully, nothing unforeseen occurred with Gordon from his and my failure to obtain more tests faster. The patient then explained how the HMO paid for all of his medical bills from the previous illness, except mine. We both laughed because my medical charge, $169 total, was the lowest he received during the entire illness. He paid my bill out-of-pocket even though I participate with Medicare, but not his HMO 2,000 miles away.

An Excessive Hospital Stay

My frail elderly patient, Spencer, had refused previously offered cancer surgery. He now had non-operable cancer and resultant kidney failure. His dear wife could no longer care for him at home. His cancer pain was uncontrolled and he was too weak to walk or care for himself. I admitted him to the hospital for blood transfusions, antibiotics and pain management. His wife agreed to take him home on the third hospital day, a Saturday, with Hospice care and some home assistace.

Spencer's children arrived at the hospital that same Saturday and insisted that he go to a nursing home for comfort care. He was too ill and weak for his wife to manage. I made arrangements that Monday. The company denied coverage for this dying man maintaining there was no need for the last two days of the hospital stay. They were on the weekend. In our community, new patients are not accepted in nursing homes on weekends. This is another market-driven solution to patients' needs.

Market-driven insurance companies, when a patient is critically ill, start an actuarial game. The longer life insurance clients live and pay on their policies, the better. But if the payout starts on an annual or monthly policy, then the sooner the clients die, the more the companies keep. The sooner the seriously ill die, the better for the HMOs and health insurance companies. In this case the patient was gracious and died less than three weeks after the "excessive" five-day hospital stay.

Skip the Hospital

Another patient of mine, eighty-nine year old Janice, was brought to the emergency room by her daughter on a Friday morning. This elderly lady was too weak to walk and could not get out of her bed. She had severe heart disease and was non-operable eight years earlier. I had treated her with multiple cardiac medications over the years. On this Friday morning, we noticed on the ER monitor the patient's heart rate was dropping to well less than forty beats per minute when normal is above sixty. I admitted her to the hospital's cardiac monitoring unit, stopped some of her medications that could be aggravating her problem and ordered physical therapy. Four days later, the patient still showed evidence of slow heart rates. I had asked the cardiologist to see her about a pacemaker, a device inserted permanently in patients to prevent slow heart rates.

On day four of her hospitalization, I received a notice from her insurance company, a Medicare HMO, stating that Janice did not meet the criteria for admission on the very first day. I was informed that I should have placed the patient in a nursing home directly from the emergency room. The market-driven motive in this case was to withhold treatment. After all, Janice was eighty-nine years old and nursing homes don't implant pacemakers.

The New York State Department of Insurance publishes an annual consumer guide on the state's twenty-one HMOs with their rankings by patient or consumer complaints. The measure is calculated by counting the number of upheld complaints divided by total premiums. The HMO that denied Janice's hospitalization ranked last, twenty-first on the list.[4]

A Lateral Transfer

While I was visiting some friends in New Jersey, one told me about his mother who has severe dementia. She was unable to recognize people and required chronic care and was at a long-term nursing home. Apparently the family did not pay the bill in time, so the nursing home sent his mother to the psychiatric hospital for evaluation. The family was not even told of her transfer until they came to visit at the home. The son immediately wired funds to the nursing home since checks were not accepted. The nursing home then agreed to accept the patient back under its care. If nursing home care was universally covered, this lateral transfer for financial reasons would not have occurred. Market-driven decisions are frequently concerned more with money than with patients.

Being Refused

This elderly patient, Harvey, required surgery for severe arthritis. Days after undergoing total joint replacement surgery, we transferred him to the rehabilitation hospital for further physical therapy and gait training. Our clinical experience shows these patients have a more successful outcome with the aggressive rehabilitation post-operatively.

For this Medicare HMO patient, things would be different. The HMO refused the rehabilitation hospitalization and insisted the patient go to a nursing home temporarily for rehabilitation. The nurses and doctors were obviously upset. We knew this patient was being treated differently solely because of his health insurance. The nurses and I tried to joke about the treatment differences, but we really knew it wasn't funny at all.

Harvey's surgeon successfully lobbied the HMO to change its decision and allow him to go to the rehabilitation hospital, but now Harvey refused, fearing the HMO would not really cover the rehabilitation hospital costs. Harvey now insisted on the nursing home and we couldn't change his mind. The situation wasn't funny to him either.

Service Not Authorized

My patient, Dan, had multiple prior heart catheterizations and obviously previous heart problems. One day, while outside of the area and walking up a flight of stairs, he had a dizzy spell and nearly passed out. Dan was hospitalized in that community and underwent several diagnostic tests. The doctors found no new medical problems and recommended an outpatient event recorder, a potentially expensive diagnostic test. When I saw Dan soon afterwards, I recommended a different but less expensive test that could also be helpful in this situation. I referred him to the local cardiologist who performs the test.

Unfortunately, Dan's insurance companies didn't agree with either of this patient's doctors. The patient had two different HMO insurances, his primary HMO was under his employer's plan and his secondary HMO coverage was under his wife's employer's plan. The local cardiologist didn't participate with the first HMO so the diagnostic test or office visit with this specialist was not covered. "The service is not authorized... refer to a different cardiologist in Gowanda, New York," they faxed. The first HMO insisted Dan see a new participating cardiologist in another community, nearly thirty miles north of our hospital. Dan resisted and tried to use his secondary insurance, his wife's and local cardiologist's HMO. The second HMO also refused coverage because he had primary insurance with the first HMO. This is the market-driven dance we encounter. Only one thing is certain in dealing with

HMOs, they will accept premium payments.

I called the new cardiologist's office for a possible appointment, but had been given the wrong number by the first HMO. I even tried to schedule the test at the other hospital, but nobody would perform the test in our community. I had to send Dan to Buffalo, two hours away by car. What if Dan passed out on that long drive? Dan was twice insured, but in reality he was not covered at all.

A *Court Order*

The conflict of profit-motivated companies and patients' needs is common to the American system. A patient, Allie, told me she could only have a medical treatment through "a court order." She explained that her worker's compensation insurance company refused to pay for therapy that her worker's compensation doctor ordered for an injury on her job. She could not afford the expensive therapy on her own, and her compensation physician did not participate with her regular health insurance.

Her lawyer who filed suit against the company told Allie there was nothing he could do to speed the court process. She would just have to wait for the court's decision as to who will pay for this therapy. This process has now been going on for three years, and Allie still has this medical problem. The terrible illness of the healthcare system in this case forced a patient to seriously delay needed therapy and obtain it through a lawsuit. With universal care the legal expenses would be zero and Allie would have been well in a short time.

Economists might say that the "market" motive of HMOs and insurance companies is to delay payment and treatment in hopes that patients will heal without treatment, pay out-of-pocket, or die.

A *Tetanus Shot*

Gerald came into my office after stepping on an old nail asking for a tetanus shot. Most people know that if they step on a rusty nail and it has been more than ten years since their last vaccination, they need a tetanus shot. I think I learned that in grade school. Our office policy required Gerald to sign a form guarenteeing payment if his insurance plan found the shot "unnecessary." His insurance would only pay for the cost of this "expensive vaccine," $16, if they found it "medically necessary." Are the insurance companies worried that providers are over-utilizing tetanus shots for their personal profit? What patient would agree to an unnecessary and sometimes painful injection?

Papers over Patients

Maybe Grace's health proxy form would not have been lost years earlier if we had computerized records. But, more importantly, I question who should make decisions for patients with advanced memory loss or severe mental incapacities.

Grace's dementia had been coming on for many years. She lived with her son, Jimmy, for a period of time. When she could no longer make it at home, Jimmy placed her in a nursing home. I remember hearing many times while visiting her how much she loved her son. She frequently called out his name, "Jimmy." But eventually her disease progressed. She was bedridden and no longer able to recognize people, talk, or even swallow food.

I assumed, as did her son, that he was her health proxy. He told me he remembered her filling out the papers many years ago because they went through a similar problem with his father. Jimmy further said to me, "Mother never would have wanted tube feedings or other aggressive treatments at this stage of her illness."

The problem arose when we could not find that Health Proxy form. The son and I agreed to treat his Mother comfortably, knowing her previous wishes. We decided tube feedings and intravenous hydration were out of the question. However, the nursing home objected. They did not have the signed form and insisted the patient have a feeding tube placed, which could possibly require surgery or hospitalization. So I hospitalized her for four days. In the hospital, nurses were able to feed her adequately; it just took a longer time to sit with the patient. We took special precautions to try to prevent an aspiration. Grace seemed comfortable and we discharged her back to the nursing home with these feeding instructions.

But Grace again stopped eating at the nursing home. Now the home feared reprisals from the New York State Health Department because we did not have that piece of paper. So against the son's wishes and my orders, the home placed an intravenous needle in the patient's arm and administered fluids.

Who are we treating here, papers or patients? Sometimes it seems we are treating papers first. I receive faxes marked "urgent" on a regular basis. Are these critical patient test results or updates on their condition? No, they are forms needing a doctor's signature to authorize payment of ambulance services already provided to sick patients. It makes me feel stupid signing them when what I should do instead is write back demanding to know what the company's priorities really are.

Sorry, No Early Refill

Another elderly patient, Edna, had many medications and pays 50% of her total $300 monthly prescription costs. Her insurance covers the rest. Edna told me how difficult and inconvenient it was for her to travel back and forth to the pharmacy for refills. Her insurance, though, will not allow a refill on a prescription if it is more than four days early. Here, the market-driven motive is cash flow. Why not let the patient have a two or three months supply of a chronic medication. No, then the insurance company would have to pay in advance. Maybe they are also concerned that the patient might die and leave some unused pills.

In this system do the companies really care or do they believe someone frail and elderly should not live? Notice here the market drive collides between two industries. The pharmaceutical companies want to sell medications. The insurance companies don't want to pay for them.

A Mail Order Rx Plan

In the system, insurance companies try to save money on patients' prescriptions. There are formularies, co-pays, restricted refills, generics only, pre-authorizations, pill cutting, no coverage, and then the ultimate, limiting what pharmacy a patient can use. Recently, one insurance company would only authorize payments if their patients used a particular pharmacy chain in our community.

One of the more obnoxious industry practices is the "three-month mail away plan" for maintenance medications. It is hard to imagine how these plans could ever be shown to save any money or improve overall quality and patient satisfaction. A patient, Larry was on a maintenance medication, *Prilosec*, costing about $100 per month. He had just received a three-month *Prilosec* shipment, when he was sent a new substitute *Prevacid*, which also costs over $100 a month. He was advised by the mail order pharmacy to stop the *Prilosec*. So the nearly $300 worth of *Prilosec* sits in his medicine cabinet at home. At the same time, Larry's thyroid prescription had not arrived by mail in time so I had to re-write a two-week prescription for him to purchase from the local pharmacy. This prescription only costs a few dollars per month generically. Why does this patient have to mail away for this "costly" medicine?

In this process, does anyone really measure the waste and the missing services? What happens if patients have questions about their medications? What happens when the patient receives a new prescription from a specialist and the local pharmacist is not aware of the current medications? Who will catch the drug incompatibility or drug-drug interaction without complete knowledge of the patient's current medications? Are there really any long-term drug savings? Have you ever tried to call and talk to a mail-order pharmacist?

Another Long Distance Pharmacist

A patient, Curry, asked me to call his mail-order pharmacy, some 2,000 miles away from Jamestown, which would not fill his prescribed medications because the medications were not on their formulary. He needed the medications and so I called the mail order pharmacy for him. I was transferred or placed on hold multiple times over a thirty-minute period. It was humorous, in a sordid way, how many different times a person can be shuffled from one voice message to another. By then I really wanted to speak with the pharmacist to express my patient's and my own frustration with their telephone system. When the actual live pharmacist answered the telephone call, he could not tell me what medications were on the formulary. He would not even try to enter other similar medications I suggested to see if they were covered. The reality is, our nations attempt to lower prescription costs places patients in serious and in some cases life-threatening situations. A recent television news report claimed error rates as high as 4% in mail-order prescriptions. I suggested the patient buy his medications locally.

On the day the local newspaper reported that Congress was considering the approval of patients buying and importing medications from foreign nations to lower their overall drug costs, I had three patients ask for samples to hold them over until their mail-order medications actually arrived to their homes. Imagine what the error rate and delays will be if patients start ordering their medications from overseas. This will not save overall healthcare costs for this nation. The patient-drug errors and the cost of care for these illnesses caused will offset any short-term drug savings.

A Same Day Rx Change

On the same day, I received requests from two different drug distribution companies. Each asked me to change my patients' medications for a cost savings. With a list of some patient's names, the first company asked me to switch my patients from *Pravachol* to *Zocor*. The second company, with a different list, asked me to switch my patients from *Zocor* to *Pravachol*. Where is the savings in healthcare costs in this nation with such absurdity? Each company had to study the patients' lists, get the prices, write the letters, make the computer entries, and check for follow-up. Some of them may have been responding to the pharmaceutical representatives and their attractive perks.

February 1, 2001

Rudolph J. Mueller, M.D.
██████████████
Jamestown, New York

Dear Doctor Mueller:

Once again, through the marvels of modern ethics, I've been duped – or should I say, "dumped"! ██████████ mail-in prescription service has discontinued their contract with ████████ My prescriptions were caught up in the resulting deluge of paperwork. Four were filled; one was mailed back (████), and one is still in their possession (████), but probably won't be filled. I have enclosed the returned script along with the form letter I received.

As all these prescriptions were just renewed in December, I am in need of new prescriptions. For convenience, pre-printed labels are enclosed to attach to your prescription slips and can be returned in the self-addressed, stamped envelope.

Thank you for your understanding.

Sincerely,

████████

████

Enclosures

A patient's letter concerning her mail-in prescription plan.

A Kick-back

A common practice in retailing is for manufacturers to offer incentives to clerks or sales persons to sell their products. A pharmacist friend told me some companies now offer these "kick-backs" to pharmacists if they can convince patients or doctors to change from one medication to another "preferred" medication. Pharmacists can receive between two and ten dollars per prescription change. This is a market-driven result that has very questionable benefit to customers or patients.

Progressive Insurance

An eighty-year old patient, Christina. had multiple medical problems and was on fairly expensive medications. I asked her if she had any prescription insurance coverage. She explained that she did but it was inadequate for her needs. The insurance covered only 10 – 15% of her prescriptions. The name of the insurance company had the word "progressive" in it. I thought "regressive" seemed more appropriate.

Christina then told me about her son who had worked for a "temporary services" company for three years. He went without health insurance during this period. He then was promised a new job with full-time work and insurance. He was good with computers and could help this new company fix their computer problem. So he changed jobs for better work and insurance. His only problem was that the new company let him go two months later. Now he was unemployed and uninsured. The mother said to me, "If I were younger, I'd be out there fighting these things." It is a dynamic of democracy that when enough people feel that way, the fight starts.

How is Your Vision?

An HMO authorized one of my patients to see an optometrist for an eye problem. The HMO optometrist prescribed non-narcotic prescription eye drops for the patient. The HMO policy denied payment to the pharmacist unless the prescription has a DEA number. Optometrists do not have DEA numbers so the HMO would not have to pay for any drug prescriptions written by optometrists. These were the same eye doctors that the HMO prefers patients see first. I had to rewrite the prescription for the patient to receive the medication.

What is the objective of this policy? It doesn't seem to be in favor of providing quality care. It costs money in salaries and office expenses to write the policies of such absurd content and then enforce them. Then doctors have to undo the harm.

A Working, Married Addict

Drug addiction is a terrible affliction, but it is treatable. I have seen one particular patient, Arthur, for many years for various medical problems and emotional distress when his drug addiction was untreated. Thankfully, Arthur sought and received drug counseling and addiction treatment. Though difficult for him and his family in so many ways, Arthur recovered his health and a life-sustaining purpose. He is now active in his church, enjoying his family and is fully employed. The insurance company covered Arthur's first year of therapy, which included an inexpensive medication and counseling. Our community however, does not offer this medication, so initially Arthur had to travel out-of-state almost daily for many weeks. I rarely saw him after this successful treatment because many of his medical problems were resolved under this current therapy.

However, the insurance company's contract did not require coverage of this medical illness after one year of therapy. Arthur and I laboriously appealed the denial of treatment, without success. He knew he could not go without treatment. He risked losing his family, his job or even his life. Arthur continued the medication and treatment costing him nearly $80 per week out-of-pocket. Had he lived in Pennsylvania, twenty-six miles away, the cost to him would have been $15 per week. Here is a $3,000 yearly cost difference in medication simply because of a patient's state of residency. This does not just border on insanity; it is insane for such policies to affect people.

However the insanity has not ended for Arthur's traumatic ordeal. He recently stopped his treatment for his addiction because of the excess cost and his lack of continuous medication insurance coverage. He sent me this letter asking me for help in dealing with his new health and

A note from Arthur

other related problems that re-entered his life after stopping his previously successful treatments. He even told me how it was cheaper for him to buy the illegal drugs, since a two-week stash costs less than a seven-day prescription. Arthur is not alone, nearly one million Americans are addicted to this illegal drug and only 20% of them are currently treated with the affordable and effective prescription medication in an addiction treatment program.[5]

And who will pay for the overall costs when many of these 800,000 Americans with addictions and lack of treatment, similar to Arthur's situation, acquire AIDS, commit crimes or face continuous unemployment? All Americans pay the heavy price of untreated drug addictions.

A Working, Married, Former Addict

I was walking through the ER when one of my patients came up to me and said, "You are not going to believe this one, Doc. I have a history of using cocaine but I've been currently drug free for three years. Unfortunately, I've had thoughts of using it again and I'm afraid I might relapse. So I called my insurance company to see if counseling was covered. It helped me in the past get off and stay off the drugs. The lady at the insurance company said I wasn't covered, unless I tested positive in the urine. So I *have to go out and use the drugs first before* I'm *covered*. Makes sense, doesn't it?" What a tragic example of incompetence in policy making. Or do the insurance executives want the addicts to commit a crime so the state will take over? That shifts the costs to the taxpayers. The societal issue never gets factored into the dynamics because the system is all about cash flow and profits.

An Insurance Company With Sick People

We read about insurance companies making and losing money in healthcare. One company lost millions in our community. The owner had multiple health insurance products. Some physicians at a meeting asked him why this health plan lost money. He responded, "All the sick people joined this plan. We had ...too good a' prescription benefit." Now didn't this owner do a good thing, making affordable medications available for sick people? However, this company didn't sell all of the health insurance plans, only the unprofitable ones.

A Profitable Insurance Company

An elderly patient, Jane, had a severe disability accompanied by chronic pain. Her physician could no longer care for her because of her complex problems and transferred her care to me. Eventually Jane's treatment worked, her pain was relatively controlled, and she regained partial mobility. Her pain medications were expensive, though. One day, her caregiver daughter came stating, "The insurance company does not want to pay for my mother's medications. I've called and written many times. They still refuse to reimburse us for over six months now. Can you help?" I had to write a letter to this company convincing them to pay for my patient's pain medications.

Now I know how some companies can remain profitable in the United States. In this case, the company denied the payment in correspondence with the patient's family, but yielded to me. Sounds like a policy for trying to avoid payments. The cost of the bureaucracy and its correspondence and my reply and negotiations will overwhelm the cost of just doing what is right in the first place. But the scheme probably works enough times to pay off, but only for the company.

A Stress Test

My patient, Mark, a veteran, had an HMO insurance plan. He also went to the VA locally because the medications cost less through the VA. Mark had multiple risk factors for heart disease. The VA doctor ordered a stress test even though he had no symptoms. The VA stress tests normally are done in Buffalo, about two hours away by car. Because of the distance and inconvenience, Mark requested the test be performed locally at the hospital. This test was reported as normal to the VA doctor. However, Mark received a bill for the services after his insurance declined coverage. They reasoned that the primary care doctor, myself, had not ordered the test. Thirty-four days after the test was performed, the family asked me to say that I ordered the test originally. The insurance company again refused coverage, stating that they needed thirty-day notification. The VA declined to pay for the test because it was not performed at the VA hospital.

This is an example of the stupidity of the transactions with which doctors must deal. Universal care would have paid for the test. The insurance companies and the HMOs have reasons not to do so. Where is the benefit to Mark, the patient in our celebrated healthcare system? This multi-layered bureaucracy creates more cost and waste for all Americans. The family had to ask me to lie so that the cost would be covered.

A recent U.S. study demonstrated that the majority of surveyed physicians use deception to secure an insurance company's coverage of medically necessary treatment.[6] Doctors in America feel they must lie or twist the truth for patients to receive necessary healthcare. It's certain that the patients and their families have to tell lies, too.

When I asked Mark why he didn't stay with the VA, he responded, "I don't trust them."

A Dishonest Supplier?

Lack of trust permeates our entire healthcare system in so many different ways. I wanted to order home oxygen for a patient, Margery, with breathing problems. I asked a home oxygen supply company to do the oxygen testing on her. I did not have the equipment in my office. They reluctantly agreed to perform the oxygen test, but preferred not to do so. "Why not perform the test? You have the equipment and also supply the oxygen; can't we keep this simple?" I asked.

The company director replied, "The patient's insurance will not authorize coverage of oxygen therapy by any company that also performed the initial qualifying oxygen test." This meant if this company does the test and finds the patient eligible for oxygen, then that same company cannot supply the treatment. Apparently the insurance company does not trust the oxygen supply companies in the United States. The director told me, "Buy the testing equipment yourself and receive $45 from the patient's insurance." I did not want to make money off of patient's tests, and I knew there were plenty of oxygen testing devices already in our community. I just wanted Margery to get the appropriate treatment including oxygen as needed.

I also see lack of trust when I order appropriate blood tests on some of my patients. An elderly patient, Mary, had obvious dementia, a disease manifested by progressive memory loss. There are many causes of dementia, and a doctor usually performs an evaluation including blood tests and x-rays before diagnosing the "exact cause." I ordered some blood work, a brain scan and wrote "dementia" on the test order forms. Medicare declined payment for the $50 blood tests because I was not more specific in the diagnosis. Needless to say, I was upset and so was she. Why should I be more specific? I had just examined Mary for the first time and made a probable diagnosis of dementia. The tests were appropriate and necessary for the patient's care! I rewrote the order as "senile dementia" and the patient's Medicare covered the tests. As doctors we have to deal with these demented rules almost daily.

You're Covered

I probably could write a whole chapter just describing the suffering this patient, Celine, had experienced in her life. She developed juvenile-onset diabetes at a young age and had a plethora of sad stories and experiences with this disease. It was sickening to both of us. Luckily we still laugh and joke about a Medicare letter she once received.

For an entire year Celine resided more in the hospital than out, suffering multiple health problems. I begged a university center to take her case and potentially save her life. "Either she makes it or not," the university doctor and I thought. The university agreed to perform both of her transplant surgeries. The university doctor said, "We'll do both of the surgeries, but only one of them is covered by Medicare, the other is experimental." Celine, her family and I were so grateful the university accepted her medical care. She had suffered so much already.

Surprisingly, she did well at surgery, until three weeks later when a major complication arose. She remained in the university hospital and intensive care unit for over a month with the entire hospital stay lasting three months. It was truly a miracle indeed when I saw Celine in my office after her life-threatening ordeal. The surgery was a success and her quality of life had improved markedly. Months later she showed me a letter from her Medicare insurance stating, we have "covered all of your medical bills except $384,000." Celine looked at me and said, "What do I do now?"

"What are they going to do, send you to collections?"

We still laugh to this day about that letter. I wish I had a copy to show. How embarrassing for our healthcare system.

Why does our healthcare system send bills to patients ill or well anyway? There are a number of potential reasons: Patients are responsible for the remaining out-of-pocket costs not covered by their insurances. Medical bills demonstrate the "actual" costs of tests and treatments patients receive. Medical bills potentially prevent fraud from providers' over-charges or erroneous claims. Medical bills prevent patients from over utilizing services because it is not "free." Medical bills incurred by patients will reduce overall healthcare costs in a market-driven healthcare system.

However, I doubt these reasons actually manifest in America. Everyone knows a medical bill is not the actual cost of the healthcare delivered. Just look at any hospital bill or doctor's office bill. The paying patients or insurance companies are frequently paying more to cover for the care of the uninsured or "under-paying" patients. Doctors and hospitals, particularly the public ones, have to cover their costs. And, clearly this country sends more medical bills to patients than any other country in the world. America also has the highest healthcare costs. Sending bills to patients is not saving money. America still faces fraud estimates of billions in taxpayer dollars per year in Medicare alone. Current patient charges and bills have not eliminated fraud. All other industrialized and democratic countries of the world provide universal healthcare and coverage for their people and do not send outrageous medical bills.

Unknown to some in the industry, medical bills can adversely affect patients' outcomes. In America, the unaffordable and outrageous medical bills may lead to unexpected and undesirable outcomes. The stories throughout this book are replete with patients unable to pay, afford, or even consider receiving their necessary medical care or treatments. I see anger, hopelessness, frustration, depression and many other feelings in so many patients in America when they face these medical bills and cost.

Too Early and Too Late

My patient, Harvey, was turning sixty-five, the magic Medicare age. He called the government office to apply for Medicare, but was told to wait until his current health insurance stopped. When he retired at sixty-five and his health insurance expired, he returned to the government office and applied for Medicare. He was told, however, it would take a few months before he could be enrolled in Medicare. Now he was temporarily uninsured.

How do I know this story? Well, Harvey missed a routine blood pressure check-up and I called him to find out why he did not show for his appointment. He explained that he was now uninsured and that he would not re-schedule his appointment until he was insured. But he promised to return, "When I'm covered." I hope nothing happens to him in between coverage like some other patients whom I have known.

Potential Death Benefits

I felt so sorry for this man. Manny had so many medical problems, including diabetes, hypertension, Parkinson's, heart failure and prior strokes. We went through a lot of illnesses together. Eventually he died at the age of eighty-eight from multiple problems.

Later I received a letter from the family asking if his death was in anyway related to an automobile accident thirteen years earlier. If so, his widow may be entitled to "widow's death benefits" by the automobile insurance company. How would I ever know the answer to that question? I only knew him for seven years, and considering his health problems, it was a miracle he made it to eighty-eight.

My experience, the medical literature, and science support the fact that the health of the nation would improve if comprehensive, quality health insurance was provided for all people in America. But we are overwhelmed with the volumes of instructions and multiple policies of hundreds of different health insurance companies and HMOs, plus government programs. Then we only cover some of the patients some of the time.

Somehow the other democratic countries of the world can provide universal healthcare for their population at a fraction of the bureaucracy and with a much smaller number of insurance companies. No other nation has for-profit HMOs.

In America, the for-profit insurance companies' primary mission is to earn profits. And multiple insurance payers only generate even greater bureaucratic requirements, which are often thrust onto the hospitals and the doctors. In my group practice I believe possibly half of our office overhead and staff time is spent in providing information to and corresponding with HMOs and insurance companies on matters of routine billing, referrals to specialists, or pre-authorizations for medications and tests. Once again, keep in mind the number of primary care doctors, over 270,000 in the U.S., and project the volume and cost of such correspondence and paper flow onto the system.

As for the HMOs, their antics have driven doctors from the profession or into early retirement. Nearly one-half of all California physicians surveyed are considering leaving the practice of medicine over the next three years in this heavily managed-care enviroment.[7] No professional with the training of a physician wants to have oversight of such incompetence with no real interest in the patients.

Healthcare is a community matter. A system with multiple insurance companies and for-profit HMOs has no rational justification. They are a cost burden of increasing proportions and their real reason for existence is to put a hand under the gush of money that flows into healthcare. The advantages of a market-driven system do not materialize and they cannot because there are none. Such a system is a sham perpetrated on the American people to keep funds flowing into private for-profit insurance accounts where they do not belong.

6: THE PROVIDERS

"The secret of the care of the patient is in caring for the patient."
Francis Weld Peabody; JAMA 1927

The honorable practice of medicine has been an art for thousands of years and has become in more recent years an honorable science. The Hippocratic Oath was taken by nearly every graduating physician in this country in the past and still is today.

I swear by Apollo the physician... that, according to my ability and judgment, I will keep this Oath.... I will follow that system of regimen which, according to my ability and judgment, I consider for the benefit of my patients, and abstain from whatever is deleterious and mischievous... Into whatever houses I enter, I will go into them for the benefit of the sick...

And the Apostle Luke, also a physician, demonstrates his profession in Luke 11:34-5:

Your eye is the lamp of your body. When your eyes are good, your whole body is full of light. But when they are bad, your whole body is full of darkness. See to it, then, that the light within you is not darkness.

For years, physicians-in-training have answered the question, "Why do you want to be a doctor?" with this simple answer, "To help people." In the United States, we now have nearly 700,000 physicians practicing this profession and, I believe, for most physicians, to the best of their abilities. Nonetheless, money, greed and bureaucracy, among other things, have grossly perverted the medical profession. For some providers in the industry hold that if a patient cannot pay you, then you do not treat him. If patients are on low paying Medicaid or HMO insurances, don't accept them. If patients are a financial risk, then don't provide care for them. If patients owe you money, send them to a collection agency, harass them or offer no return appointments. Also don't forget to take advantage of the numerous perks offered by drug companies!

What has happened to this honorable profession? At what price with what effect on patients? And at whose injustice and at what price? When I told a colleague I was writing this book, he said, "You're writing about the dark side of medicine." Here are some examples just in the last two years.

You Have the Money, Don't you?

I was called away from a patient in the examination room by another patient's urgent phone call. It was from Helen who was experiencing major depression and suicidal thoughts, whom I had seen in the office a few days earlier. During that office visit I realized her treatment was not working, and I phoned a specialist asking for help. This specialist agreed to see her as soon as possible but I am not sure of what subsequently happened.

As Helen explained to me, she called the specialist for an appointment, but was told, "in six weeks." Then she was asked by the specialist, "And you have the money to pay me, don't you? I have to get paid, you know." I was shocked. I felt it was another traumatic blow to her chances of recovery. Obviously this patient was now in more despair and cried out to me over the phone, "What do I do now?"

"I'll call the specialist back and I'm sure we'll get you seen," I wishfully explained.

This patient did get seen, but in the county's psychiatric clinic and not in the physician's private office. And I knew she even had the money to pay. Why? Two years earlier, an insurance company selling long-term insurance denied coverage to Helen even at a premium of $6,000 per year. I remember then thinking, "How could anyone afford long-term health insurance at that cost?" She was willing to pay the premium, but the company thought she was too great a risk for them to take.

She told me then, "I want to buy nursing home insurance so I won't burden my family in the future." I remember thinking to myself, "Who would ever want to buy nursing home insurance? No one wants to go to a nursing home." Here was a patient willing to pay $6,000 per year for nursing home insurance so she surely had enough money for the specialist's private office. Something went wrong in this patient-doctor encounter. The specialist convinced himself that he might not be paid for his services so off to the county mental health clinic she went.

It Pays Not to Participate

Another elderly patient of mine, Jeannette, wanted to see a specialist in the community because of ongoing medical problems. When she called the specialist's office for an appointment, she was told to "bring in $208" for the initial examination by the doctor. The specialist was a non-participating doctor with Medicare. The patient decided instead to go out of town for her specialty care and see a doctor in Cleveland, only a three-hour drive each way.

Did He Have To Get Rich Over Night?

I performed a cancer-screening test on Fred and found a possible abnormality. He required a referral to a specialist but no one in this specialty practiced within thirty miles of our community or participated with his HMO. While his HMO insurance restricted patients to "only participating doctors," a New York State "thirty minute, thirty mile" rule allowed Fred to see a local specialist. This rule was another stopgap measure in New York State to allow patients adequate access to specialists.

Fred did have an abnormality, and the test thankfully enabled the problem to be corrected. But he returned to me complaining of the bills he received from the doctor and the hospital. I told him, "Don't worry, your insurance will cover it. How much was it anyway?"

"The bill is $2,600 split into $1,600 for the doctor and $1,000 for the hospital. And it only took them forty minutes to do the test. The doctor even had ten to twelve other patients lined up in a row that day. I know the doctor had to go to school but did he have to get rich overnight?"

I tried to explain that the equipment was expensive, nearly $10,000 and the test usually costs $1,000. At least that is what I have been told. "I understand the equipment costs a lot, but did I have to buy it myself?" he commented. I apologized for the bills and tried to reassure him. What do patients without insurance do with bills like these? This assumes they have the tests.

Simple for Whom

A recently initiated national physician healthcare plan had the word "simple" in its title. This plan was tailored to those patients without insurance and offered outpatient physician visits at "reduced fees" of "30%-50%" of routine charges. Additional benefits to the doctor and patient included no paperwork or insurance forms to file. All patients had to do was join the plan for a minimal amount and then pay cash or use a credit card at the time of physician service. Physicians could "afford" to offer these reduced fees because of reduced administrative costs and increased cash flow. Patients were encouraged to still purchase catastrophic health insurance or an MSA to "protect themselves" financially during times of costly and prolonged illness.

What struck me as most humorous about the "simple" plan was the "reduced fees." Physician office visits were $35 for ten minutes, $65 for twenty minutes and $95 for sixty minutes. Assuming the physician has thirty hours a week of direct face-to-face patient contact, a participating physician may collect nearly $200 per hour and possibly up to $300,000 per year. That doesn't include any other income from other sources or any other charges the patients may face. For the physician, it offers no red tape or forms to file and payment up-front. Now that is a "simple" plan, simple for the doctor assuming the patients can afford the fees.

Here is another true story: I received a phone call from a medical consultant describing a plan to help the uninsured in western New York. A group of physicians agreed to treat uninsured patients for cash or credit card at the time of service with fees up to 115% of Medicare. "That's big of the physicians!" I exclaimed jokingly. That is nearly $150-200 per hour cash up-front for a primary care physician and that includes no insurance forms to complete. It seemed like another good deal for the physicians, but what about the patients?

What happens to the patient who does not have the money at the time they need care or can't afford even these reduced fees? What happens to the patient in the emergency room or in the hospital? Do physicians collect money from patients lying in bed before examining them? And how do patients pay for their prescriptions? Maybe pharmacists will give them a "simple" break on their charges.

The Patient's Fault

When in doubt about, or unwilling to change a broken healthcare system, one can always blame the patient. The American Medical Association Foundation, the philanthropic arm of the AMA, believes it may have discovered a root cause of many medical errors: *patients themselves*![1] The AMA and other physician groups don't endorse national health insurance, such as Medicare-for-all. Their major objection may be related to money and their fear of reduced physician incomes.

In 1999, the average U.S. primary care physician's yearly income was $143,970 while a specialist's was $245,910. Their average charges or "productivity" increased by 11.6% to $374,702 for primary care and 8.5% to $785,900 for specialty care from the year before. But the collection of gross charges by physicians has steadily declined over the past twenty years from an average of 88.8% in 1980 to 67.7% in 1999. To maintain their incomes, with continual rising overhead and reduced collections, physicians have had to work harder by seeing more patients per hour or working more hours overall. Some have expanded potential income-generating sources by providing office-based diagnostic and surgical services, alternative medical treatments, clinical

research, and lecturing for drug companies. Some physician incomes fell in
1999, but most continued to climb and out-pace inflation.[2]

American physicians are by far the highest paid in the world. Canadian
physicians have lower incomes despite significantly lower billing and office
overhead costs compared to their American counterparts. For example, U.S.
physicians incur $328 per capita more overhead costs than the Canadian
physicians.[3] Some U.S. physicians fear a Canadian type system would significantly reduce their personal incomes. The truth is U.S. physicians are only
collecting two-thirds of their current charges, and if their bureaucracy were
reduced to Canadian equivalents, U.S. physicians could increase their net
income by more than $100,000 per year.[4]

I am not asking for physicians to be paid more money than they are
now. But there is tremendous waste and bureaucracy in the current system.
A single-payer Canadian (or other OECD nation) model program could lower
overall physician overhead and charges significantly, while still maintaining
high incomes. Currently U.S. physician incomes are in the top 5% of the
entire population.[5] I'm certain that most people would agree that their doctors should be paid well and appreciate the time and sacrifice these professionals have, and will continue, to put forth for their patients. Most
physicians I know graduated at or near the top of their high school and college classes and earned many honors in rigorous academics. Americans
want the best doctors for their families and themselves. However, there may
be other factors that also account for the high costs associated with U.S.
physicians.

Medical Education Cost

In 1997, the average yearly tuition and fees for private medical schools averaged $24,930, and the average debt for a four-year medical education for all
medical students was $80,462. Some students can accumulate debts well
over $200,000 by the time of their graduation.[6] Since 1984, U.S. physician
salaries have increased by 68% but the corresponding debt level at gradua-
tion has increased by 248%. More than half of all borrowing over the past
three decades for medical students has occurred since 1990.[7]

Unfortunately large medical student debt does influence future doctors'
career decisions. One survey of medical students showed that nearly 50% of
all students wanted to pursue careers as primary care physicians but those
facing higher debts instead chose subspecialty careers and the potential,
future higher incomes. In turn, only 29% chose primary care fields.

The U.S. also needs more minorities in the profession. African-
Americans account for 15% of the total U.S. population, but are well under
10% of the enrolled population in U.S. medical schools over the past two

decades.[8] I believe the necessary education debt and high costs prevent many poor and minority students from pursuing medical degrees.

Surprisingly, U.S. medical student tuition and fees pay very little in comparison to the overall U.S. medical school revenues. In 1997-1998, 2.8% of the entire revenue of public medical schools and 5.1% of private medical schools revenues came from tuition and fees, totaling $1.5 billion.[9] Many of the wealthy industrialized OECD nations provide students "free" medical education, leaving these future doctors relatively debt-free compared to their American counterparts. Physician collections in this nation are 20% of the total healthcare dollars and reach well over $200 billion per year. How much of America's high physician charges and incomes are related to their medical education debt relative to the other OECD physicians over time?

I believe America should consider paying for all of the medical school education costs of the students. The $1.5 billion extra investment per year would lead to more doctors going into primary care and/or fields of their actual first choice, lower the life-time physician medical education debt and increase the number of minority and overall medical student applications. These are all laudable goals for a sound healthcare delivery system.

I am thankful and grateful that my father and brother paid for my medical education. If I had a $200,000 medical education debt, would I have pursued my current career in general internal medicine and geriatrics? I hope so, but I did not have to face those difficult financial decisions. High medical education debt is not the only hurdle or obstacle U.S. physicians must face and overcome.

Malpractice Fear, Plaintiff Lawyers and Reality

At the dawn of the new millennium, doctors and other providers face aggressive and influential external forces. One cannot discuss physicians without mentioning lawyers and malpractice fears. Telephone books, billboards and newspaper advertisements are replete with plaintiff lawyers asking, "Have you been injured lately?"

Sometimes the injuries are legitimate claims of malpractice, but frequently they aren't. American physicians practice the most defensive medicine in the world and everyone in America is paying for the additional costs.

My heart was saddened when I read the front page headlines of a local newspaper reporting the enormous malpractice judgment against a local colleague and the hospital. The median settlement in America in 1999 was over $500,000 per case, but the jury delivered a prize of $20 million in this case.[10] This involved a man presenting to the emergency room with a prior history of kidney stones and back pain. According to the newspaper account, it took five hours to diagnose a ruptured aneurysm. The patient required emergency surgery and eventually lost both legs secondary to severe ischemia from the "delayed diagnosis."

What surprised me in this case was the size of the jury award, considering the patient's eventual outcome. This patient presented with an acute dissecting aneurysm, which has a grave prognosis and extremely high mortality rate. But this patient survived his brush with mortality. I am told the plaintiff's attorney also declined settling this case out of court. A recent appeal by the defense to a judge helped lower the judgment but unfortunately the new amount was still well above that covered by insurance. The hospital and physician each had $2 million of malpractice protection. I wonder if the patient, his family and the plaintiff's attorney will go after the assets of the now retired doctor and the hospital next.

And what about this physician, who was and still is respected in our community? This doctor volunteered in Africa and performed missionary work for many years at little or no pay. Every doctor in our community knows how this physician has made a positive difference in so many patients' lives.

One in seven doctors and one in eight dentists in 1990 have had a liability judgment or settlement and I'm sure those figures are only climbing. I do not know any practicing physicians personally in this country who have not been named in a malpractice lawsuit at one time in their career. But I have never met or seen any physician or nurse who purposely tried to harm a patient, either. Physicians, dentists, and nurses are not God but human beings, who are capable of making errors.

It is also inevitable that patients or families are angry or upset with poor or unexpected medical outcomes. Others may have no other means of further treatments or care without litigation. American physicians practice the most defensive medicine in the world. Doctors commonly over test and over treat patients for fear of malpractice.

The day prior to scheduled surgery, I read a *Newsweek* article titled, "Mediation Before Malpractice Suits?" I was waiting for my (probably unnecessary) pre-operative electrocardiogram. The authors mentioned "alternative dispute resolution" before litigation. "Our experience suggests that when patients and providers work out their differences face to face in a non adversarial forum, they generate better solutions to problems. Patients gain more influence over the healthcare system and providers emerge with a stronger commitment to making it work." The article went on to say, "Patients have three main desires. First, they want a full explanation of what occurred and why. Second, they want an acknowledgment or apology from the caregiver. And third, they want to know what steps were taken to ensure that what happened to them would not happen to someone else."

If not mediation and alternative dispute resolution, then why not "no-fault" insurance? In New York we have mandatory "no-fault" automobile insurance. Why not mandatory health insurance for human beings and "no-fault" malpractice insurance for their providers? A recent article suggests implementing a no-fault compensation system for medical injuries in the U.S. The estimate of such a no-fault program for medical injuries would not exceed the current costs of malpractice insurance today.[11]

There are other unfortunate side effects of the plaintiff bar in medicine. Some patients rely on publicly funded health clinics for their preventive or primary healthcare needs. Unfortunately, in our community, and possibly other communities, the "free" clinic offered two times a year had been discontinued. Supposedly, the clinic managers feared potential liability risks from uninsured patients. A clinic volunteer nurse explained management's decision. Uninsured patients may have abnormal cancer screening tests, but no insurance or doctor with whom to do a follow-up. Such a patient's cancer may go untreated and lead to potential liability risks for the clinic. So it is safer for the clinic to not screen the uninsured patients.

Is this what it means to live in America? Don't provide charity care because of your liability risks!

Litigation and malpractice fears and reality hurt more than just the injured parties. The effects ripple through the entire system with obvious costly and adverse outcomes. I do not assert that errors and mistakes don't occur in medicine, but surely we can find a better way to prevent future mistakes and compensate the injured fairly.

War on Fraud

The "war" on fraud is real to many providers with the recent wave of Medicare fraud investigations by the government. An emergency room physician told me, "I feel like a criminal every day." He explained how he feared federal agents would come "marching in with guns drawn" to examine his billing records. Busy doctors who know they make mistakes in their records are afraid of overly aggressive scrutiny. I talked to him about the problems of the uninsured and underinsured. He quickly opposed any universal health insurance program; "I didn't go into medicine to be a minister."

Another colleague, a surgeon, complained about the medical chart documentation required to avoid potential fraud investigations. There is little argument that the current documentation requirements are too cumbersome, and frequently irrelevant to quality medical care. In the dialog that started, I suggested to this surgeon that maybe physicians should be paid according to the time they spend with the actual patient. A recent article in a leading medical journal proposed such an alternative to the existing bureaucratic nightmare that nearly all U.S. physicians face.[12]

Time, meaning minutes spent with a patient, is a number that would require less documentation and allow patients more opportunities to recognize discrepancies in billing codes. Many professionals are paid according to their time of service; accountants, lawyers and mechanics to name a few. If they overstate their time of services performed, customers immediately know. This surgeon objected to time and its relation to charges arguing, "If I can perform surgery faster than another surgeon, should I not be able to make more money?" I don't pretend to know all the answers to physician's payment methods, but do we really want physicians reading x-rays, operating or examining patients as quickly as possible?

Fraud unfortunately does occur in the health profession. I remember testifying against a local pharmacist who defrauded the government of millions of dollars in false prescription claims. I was angry when the pharmacist's defense lawyer questioned me on all the prescriptions that were filed fraudulently in my name to different government insurance programs. "Maybe you don't remember writing those prescriptions," the attorney suggested to me. Some of the medications were obviously contraindicated in my patients. And, all of the fraudulent claims were expensive medications.

This example and other forms of true fraud by providers and physicians are uncommon. But the fear in all providers is real and universal. A simple, inclusive system with a rational funding mechanism likely would lead to less fraud. Fraud investigations are uncommon in other countries of the world with universal healthcare systems. I find it sad when physicians not only fear patients because of potentially future litigation, but also fear their government over potential complex, non-clinical documentation issues.

Another benefit a single-payer payment system would provide is the greater risks a perpetrator of fraud would incur. Presently, providers may commit fraud, be prosecuted and continue to practice, not only in different states but also the same state with different insurance companies. With a single-payer system, a repeated fraud offender would have no other options but to leave the system all together. I doubt more providers would be willing to take those risks in a single-payer system compared to our current fragmented system. Fear of fraud investigations and lawsuits are not the only concerns on the minds of American doctors.

Loss of Freedom

Possibly the most profound external effect on the doctors and other providers may be the false perceptions generated by their own lobbies. The lobbies promote the benefits of the market-driven concept while simultaneously oppose the results of the market. Some may argue, "Where are the good old days?"

The lobbies and some physician colleagues argue against universal healthcare and predominant government funding because they fear their loss of liberty and freedom to practice medicine. They probably fear that a single-payer system would reduce their incomes. The lobbies point to various governmental interferences such as fraud investigations, burdensome adminstration, guidelines and international healthcare problems as proof of their government's lack of competence to deliver a national program. There is confusion in the medical profession about what the national and societal goals should be for all Americans.

The American people, in my judgment, will not allow this system of multi-level barriers to continue blocking their medical needs. People seem unaware of the roadblocks and obstacles, only to recognize them when they or their family members seek treatment in the sick system. In America, the insurance company and HMO reviewers are in the examining rooms and surgical suites, frequently telling doctors and patients what they can and cannot do. The right system, modeled after some of the best features in the OECD nations health programs, will get the bureaucrats out and allow all patients to come in and receive the best possible care by their doctors and hospitals.

A national healthcare program in the U.S. can deliver more freedom to patients, doctors, hospitals, and other providers if based on these fundamental principles. The program must be publicly accountable, publicly financed, locally administered and provide quality, accessible, affordable, comprehensive care for all people. Patients must have the freedom to choose their doctor, hospital or other providers. Providers must have the freedom to practice medicine to the best of their abilities.

The confusion about this program leads me to feel like a spy when I walk into the hospital medical staff lounge. I place medical articles and editorials on the bulletin board or table for other physicians to read. It is what happens to these articles next that makes me feel as if I'm a stranger in a strange land.

For example, one article evaluated patients' outcomes and their relationship to out-of-pocket costs. This study clearly showed that elderly or poor patients with higher out-of-pocket costs had higher mortality rates when all other clinical factors were equal.[13] But someone removed the article from the medical staff bulletin board within three days, and I doubt it was the cleaning lady.

I placed an editorial, written by two female physicians, supporting universal health insurance and a single-payer system in the lounge. This expounded on the virtues and health benefits to all people but the article lasted only seven days before disappearing.[14] I have posted other medical articles that have been mysteriously covered up including an editorial, "Is U.S. Healthcare Really the Best?" The editorial only confirmed the many facts and reasons why we do not have the best care in the world.[15] I guess the truth hurts and it is important to cover it up.

Sometimes articles have been defaced with derogatory comments such as an article from the AMN*ews*, titled "Not-in Practice Guidelines."[16] It contained an interview and picture with an ethicist supporting the use of practice guidelines, a controversial subject for some physicians. This ethicist questioned whether it was ethical for doctors not to use current standards or guidelines for most patients. Obscene comments were written above the ethicist's picture in less than ten hours.

Are Physicians Slaves?

One article placed on this same medical staff board stated, "Physicians are slaves."

Surprisingly this article remained uncovered and was not removed for over six months. I often wonder, "If the average U.S. physician can earn well over $160,000 per year, live or practice in just about any place he wishes, enjoy better health and healthcare access, face little unemployment, exactly how are physicians slaves?" And if these 700,000 American physicians are slaves, what does that make the sick people, the patients for whom physicians supposedly work and care? Are not the patients who are dependent on medications, dialysis machines and our medical treatments also slaves? Actually, who is the master, and who is the slave? And what about police officers, firemen, nurses, teachers, judges, and other public servants? Are they slaves, too? I find the connection of slavery embarrassing to the profession.

Gregg Esterbrook once wrote for *Newsweek*, "The medical mind is a complex arena. Within it an ethic of service is at war with a craving for gain. Most occupations make no pretense of an obligation to human kindness. But physicians must vow to place others above themselves, and it is a vow most doctors struggle to honor. Those who lose the conflict between their better and lesser natures may descend into self-pity."[17]

Racism

Unfortunately, racism still thrives, even in the healthcare system. Studies have clearly shown the Hispanic and African-American people are less insured and have higher mortality and morbidity rates compared to the non-Hispanic white population. At lunch with a colleague one day we discussed the problems of the uninsured, especially among minority populations. The Hispanic community was growing in our city. The 2000 census reports that the U.S. has over 35 million Hispanic-Americans or 12.5% of the entire population.[18]

Our community includes a large Puerto Rican immigrant population and may be perceived by others as a cause of high Medicaid costs. I was surprised when a physician said, "The Puerto Ricans are lazy and smell." It was sad to hear such a comment from an educated community leader, let alone a physician. I have heard nearly 20% of all medications taken by U.S. patients are manufactured in Puerto Rico.

I then went home and told my senior neighbor, who has lived in our community for many years, about the physician's comments. My neighbor responded, "That's the same thing they said about the Italians in the 1950s." He went on to observe how different groups of human beings have been victims of prejudice for years in America. We too soon forget nearly every person in this country is an immigrant or has had previous family members who were immigrants at some time in history.

I decided to ask the next Puerto Rican patient in my office about his life and why he came to the United States. In came seventy-year old Pietro, with bilateral below knee amputations from multiple diabetic complications.

"When did you come to the U.S.?" I asked him.

"In 1956," Pietro answered.

"Why," I asked?

"I could make better money in the U.S. for my family," he responded. He never went to college, but he worked hard up until the age of sixty-five and then retired. Prior to his retirement, he had to wrestle with his diabetic health problems for many years.

Now he proudly showed me his family pictures in his wallet. His son went to college and "got a good job" in aviation. "Makes over $50,000 per year," he said. Then with a big proud smile, he added, "Here are my grandchildren. Aren't they wonderful?" It seemed like the American Dream had come true for this patient's family.

A recent editorial in a leading medical journal, "Racial Injustice in Healthcare" expanded on the unfortunate truth that racism still exists, even in medicine.[19] The authors cited numerous medical studies showing how people of color are treated differently than caucasians in a democratic society. The authors state, "We believe the common thread in these findings is a subtle form of racial bias on the part of medical care providers. The level and extent of this problem are unknown, but it is real and potentially harmful, even though predominantly unintentional. Americans, we believe, perceive, value, and behave toward one another through a lens of race. This lens can create false assumptions that result in unintended but serious harm to members of minority groups—especially those who are powerless and vulnerable." The authors conclude with, "Physicians, as well as pharmacists, police officers, and others, must learn to see people not through the lens of race but instead as the individual persons they are. Appropriate judgments and actions in medicine and in society at large will follow."

The Best Doctors

I placed another medical study, involving over 2,000 medical students, residents, fellows, academic faculty, residency program directors and deans of medical schools, in the medical lounge. This random survey examined these physicians' attitudes towards managed care. When asked their preference for an overall type of system, 57% favored a universal coverage, single-payer system over a fee-for-service or managed care market-based system.[20]

I called the study's author for a breakdown among the groups surveyed. When the physicians-in-training were removed from the above figures, I was even more surprised. Now 69% of over 1,000 randomly selected academic physicians favored a universal coverage, single-payer system over the present systems.[21]

When I told another colleague that "the best" U.S. physicians, academic physicians, now favored universal coverage, single-payer over our current system, he objected saying, "No, Rudy, we're the best doctors."

This same physician refuses to see his own patients in nursing homes. His excuse, "The nursing home medical directors are paid more" than he would be for his services and continued care. I guess $50–$70 is not enough to see your own patient every one to two months. I always believed general internal medicine physicians practiced adult medicine and would care for their patients from the beginning of adulthood until the end of their lives, if possible. I think some physicians feel it is too inconvenient to travel ten minutes one-way to see their patients in a nursing home. Other doctors think about how inconvenient it is for the patient to leave his real home to enter a nursing home and obtain a new doctor.

Inconvenience may have explained this next occurrence or perhaps it was something else. One of my patients was also seeing a specialist, but was not completely satisfied with his care. He wanted a second opinion and called the specialist's office for a referral. The specialist's nurse called him back and said, "The doctor doesn't give referrals." Was it too much inconvenience or too much pride for the doctor?

The patient, however, after all is the key matter, but this concept gets lost along the way sometimes. I believe these examples demonstrate signs of a sickness permeating the U.S. medical profession. Unfortunately, the present system mocks professionalism. The results are anger, denial, and loss of hope and professionalism for some physicians.

Computers and Big Brother

My neighbor's daughter picked up some medication for a chronic medical problem at the pharmacy. She had insurance and did not need samples. Soon after she started taking the refilled medications, though, she developed new neurological problems. Was it multiple sclerosis or a brain tumor? The doctors, parents and patient feared the worst. Multiple tests and two brain MRIs failed to make the diagnosis. Luckily, the treating physician examined the recently filled prescription and tested the pills. They were the wrong medication. She was taking a toxic dose of the mistaken drug, a similar color and size of her previous medication tablets. She recovered, thankfully, but this demonstrates an event in medicine similar to the airline industry's, "near miss." Would a computerized drug-dispensing unit tied into her medical records have prevented this error? The answer is "probably."

Some recent studies have demonstrated how computers can protect patients from human error. Unfortunately, the healthcare industry will probably be the last to fully embrace computers in direct patient care.

Some people fear an electronic medical record because of loss of personal privacy and "Big Brother." These are reasonable concerns and issues, but what about patient safety and quality medical care? Would you really fly an airline that didn't fully use computers? Do you fear your loss of privacy and "Big Brother" when you use your credit card for your everyday purchases or travel destinations?

I received a fax in my office. The night before, one of my patients had been in the emergency room with pneumonia. The treating emergency room physician unintentionally ordered an antibiotic to which the patient was allergic. At the time, the patient did not remember the allergy and the emergency room did not have access to my office records. Neither the emergency room nor my office clinical records are computerized, but both locations have sophisticated computerized billing systems! Luckily, this patient had no significant reaction. It was just another "near miss."

I think patients sometimes assume their doctor has all the information in front of him and knows how other doctors have treated them. Even if doctors take thorough histories and review available information, much important information sometimes can slip through the cracks and lead to less than desirable patient outcomes. It is time for our healthcare system to more fully utilize computerized medical records in direct patient care instead of concentrating on computerized billing systems. The technology is available as evidenced by the sophisticated systems pharmacies and pharmaceutical companies utilize compared to the typical physician's office, hospital, or emergency room. Of course, all computerized systems must protect patient confidentiality.

The Hospital Pressures

The market-driven system creates nightmares for the hospitals, too. The multiple payers and reviewers required by the market-driven system are enough to frustrate and demoralize just about anybody or any institution. I am optimistically surprised at how some hospital administrators, nurses and other professionals can maintain their good humor and cheerfully try their best every day. There are many who still want to devote their lives to the service of all patients at all levels. But many have left hospitals, while still others come to work frustrated with a system that seems unjust, uncaring, and unchangeable.

Some hospitals are well managed. Most are public, not-for-profit institutions dependent on good administrators coordinating the services and handling chronic financial difficulties. The multiple payers lead to confusion in patient charges followed by misunderstandings and uncertainties. Sometimes the hospitals are blamed for overcharges. All hospitals develop yearly budgets, but most are never quite sure whether the monies will be there in the end.

I admitted Tom to the hospital because he was failing from multiple problems. The specialist and I did various tests and adjusted medications as an outpatient without success. The CAT scans and lab tests showed no obvious reason for his worsening condition. The patient belonged to a Medicare HMO where the hospital is reimbursed on a per diem basis instead of a Diagnosis Related Group (DRG), payment method. We scheduled a biopsy for Friday, but a conflict in scheduling occurred, and the test was moved to Monday morning. (I later learned biopsies were not performed on weekends.) We had no more new treatments to offer Tom, and so I ordered an Alternate Level of Care, (ALC) for that Saturday. Tom and his wife wanted him to remain in the hospital until after the biopsy, which was fine with me. The biopsy was performed on Monday, and the patient was discharged that same day. Two days later, the biopsy showed an aggressive and untreatable cancer. I consulted with Hospice and Tom died at home four weeks later.

Hospice covers all necessary treatments for qualified patients and is funded by the government. Hospice patients and families receive no medical bills. According to a Hospice nurse in our community, the median stay in Hospice is less than two weeks. The vast majority of Americans who die are not in Hospice care. Nearly 80% of deaths occur in the Medicare population, but Medicare fails to cover the majority of these end of life medical costs. Thirty-nine percent of terminally ill patients reported moderate to severe cost-related problems at the end of life in the U.S.[22]

Months later I was called by the hospital coding department asking if I would change the hospital orders I had previously written for Tom. I was asked to remove the ALC order I had written and say he needed two more days, Saturday and Sunday, for inpatient care. The hospital would then be reimbursed $600 per day at a per diem rate, instead of $150 per day at an ALC rate, for two additional days. I declined to change the order and told the caller, "You do not have to worry about Tom costing the hospital any more money. He died."

I understand why hospitals in the U.S. must do these things to remain financially solvent. Some studies show the for-profit hospitals are even more aggressive and have inflated or up-coded patient DRGs. When some not-for-profit hospitals are losing money in a market-driven system, they start acting like for-profit hospitals. The local hospital in my community lost $6 million in 1998 after the 1997 Balanced Budget Act took effect. At the same time, it had $40 million of unpaid charges. Just about every hospital in New York State has lost money now or in the recent past. Four hospitals closed in Cleveland, Ohio, in 1999 alone, and two were teaching institutions. The healthcare lobbies would have us believe hospitals only close in Canada.

The market-driven system with its related propaganda, wreaks havoc on the profession of medicine and the hospitals. Theoretically, the drive for profit gives the patients superior value. The problem is that the competition is imperfect, and patients frequently lack choice, and in true emergencies, cannot and should not shop around for their care. Hospitals and insurance companies already know the competitors' prices and most hospitals within a region are paid similar rates for similar conditions under DRGs. Some of my colleagues oppose a single-payer system. And yet, when they negotiate with insurance companies for their professional charges, doctors use Medicare fees as the base standard. When doctors negotiate rates significantly higher than Medicare, they are happy. But when the rates fall below Medicare, they feel underpaid and overworked.

Greed

I guess it comes down to the basics in a money-driven health system. Which is first, profits or patients? Maybe the article placed in the doctor's lounge, "Greed Versus Compassion," will help to clarify the issue.[23] The author asked, "What's the noblest of human motivations? For me, the noblest of human motivations is greed. By greed I mean being only or mostly concerned with getting the most one can for oneself and not necessarily concerned about the welfare of others." The author went on to further explain himself, and later re-stated, "Greed promotes other wonderful outcomes." The article concluded: "While human motivations, such as charity, love, or concern for others are important and salutary, they are nowhere nearly as important as people's desire to have more for themselves. We all know that, but we pretend

it is not so. That unwillingness to acknowledge personal greed as vital
to human welfare, and instead view it as disapproval, makes us easy prey
to charlatans and quacks who'd take away our liberties in the name of
combating greed."

Many others in the profession feel differently. Dr. Tinslay Harrison, a
physician, wrote more than forty years ago: "No greater opportunity, responsibility or obligation can fall to the lot of a human being than to become a
physician. In the care of the suffering he needs technical skill, scientific
knowledge, and human understanding. He who uses these with courage,
with humility and with wisdom will provide a unique service for his fellow
man and will build an enduring edifice of character within himself. The physician should ask of his destiny no more than this. He should be content with
no less."[24]

Some people see and feel that greed is one of man's most dangerous
human behaviors. Greed has brought down many "great" people, many corporations and more than a few societies.

I was having breakfast one day in the hospital when the business manager of a local medical group practice joined the conversation. The nation's
healthcare system, the problems and potential solutions came up in the conversation. He commented, "The system won't change. You might as well
make as much money as you can!" I wondered how many other people in the
industry felt that way.

It seems that some physicians and other providers have lost their focus
along the way. I really believe that all providers in the industry need to carefully consider Peabody's words, "The secret of the care of the patient is in
caring for the patient." When this happens, the rest of America's healthcare
woes will fall by the wayside.

What would happen to civilization and the medical profession if our
dominating motive were greed? Regrettably, we may now be observing this
slow disintegration. Other nations have, however demonstrated that the disease is reversible.

My father, a physician, always told me, "Don't worry about money. Find
something you love doing, and the money will take care of itself." And I still
love practicing medicine and being a physician.

7: THE OTHER HEALTHCARE SYSTEMS

"It is essential to liberty that the government in general should make a common interest with the people."

James Madison

Evaluating the healthcare systems and policies of other nations is important in determining the strong and weak points of our own system. As mentioned, in every other industrialized democratic country of the world, healthcare is a validated human right. The intention of those governments is to provide for the well-being and dignity of individuals of every economic class. In the United States, however, there is a large healthcare underclass. As reported earlier, an OECD survey showed that only 45% of Americans have guaranteed health insurance.[1]

Most OECD countries guarantee health insurance for nearly 100% of their population, while realizing the importance of the caregivers (doctors, nurses, and hospitals) and pharmaceutical companies. It is in these countries' experiences that we should seek a structure for healthcare for the United States. All that is British in healthcare is not necessarily bad. All that is French is not necessarily good.

For the elite of America and the fully insured, the treatment available may be the best in the world. But the system fails so many others and leaves a massive underclass of patients. Continuing our present system is far too expensive and incredibly unjust.

Otto von Bismarck inaugurated the first healthcare program in the world for German citizens in the newly unified nation in 1883 as part of an embryonic social contract. Starting in the 1940s and continuing through the 1970s, European countries provided and guaranteed a basic level of universal care to their citizens.[2] For virtually all Europeans, healthcare delivery to the patient is based on medical need.

These countries, that provide universal healthcare coverage, have dramatically lower overall costs. Their people enjoy higher life expectancy, more years without disability, lower infant mortality rates, and greater general patient satisfaction compared to the United States.[3] The U.S. continues to demonstrate the mediocre overall health of its people. I believe this is unsatisfactory for this great nation. According to a 1998 Commonwealth Fund Survey, 28% of Americans found it "extremely," "very," or "somewhat difficult" to get medical care when needed compared to 21% in Canada and 15% in Australia and Great Britain. Americans had six physician visits per year per capita compared to 6.5 in Germany and France, 6.6 in Australia and 6.8 in Canada. In 1997, Americans had the shortest hospital stays compared to all OECD countries at 7.3 hospital days compared to 9.8 in Great Britain, 8.4 in Canada, 10.0 in France and Australia, and 12.5 in Germany. Recently, I saw one of my patients after he had heart bypass surgery and he told me his hospital stay was only three and a half days. Thankfully, he did well; others have not.

According to a recent study, bypass patients have seen significantly shorter hospital stays averaging 5.4 in 1998 versus 9.2 days in 1990. Unfortunately, in 1998 patients were ten times more likely to be readmitted and 15 times more likely to be transferred to an extended care facility with an average length of stay being 10.6 days.[4]

In Canada, the cost of healthcare to families of different incomes is skewed so that the wealthier share more of the burden. In the United States that skew is reversed. The poor pay more for care as a percentage of income.[5] Even in countries with universal care, the poor continue to have worse outcomes compared to the rich. This disparity between rich and poor is profound. Part of the disparity is the economic and societal pressures placed on the poor, sick patients.

In a society with a large income gap between the rich and the poor, citizens die at a higher rate compared to people living in more equitable societies. Some refer to and measure this gap as the "Robin Hood index" which relates to the size of income differences between the rich and the poor. Figure Five demonstrates the relationship between income inequality in individual states versus overall mortality.[6] This income gap and its relationship to overall mortality of a population have also been demonstrated in other studies.[7]

In the U.S., the wealthiest nation in the world in GDP per capita at purchasing power parity, there is a wide and continually growing gap between the rich and the poor. From 1960 to 1986 overall mortality rates fell, but more significantly for the rich and well educated, and less so for the poor and less-educated Americans.[8] Then the economic boom in the 1990s supposedly benefited all Americans, but most of the significant gains went to those in the top 20%. Those in the middle groups may actually have become worse off

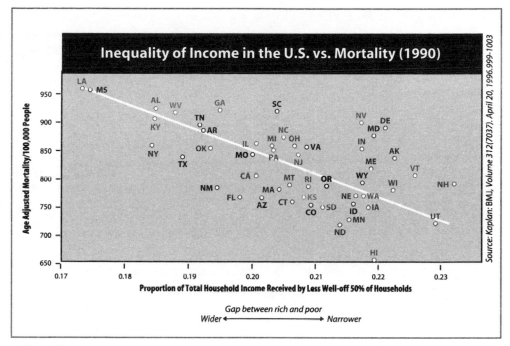

Figure Five

financially during those prosperous times.[9] Another report from a 1999 Public Policy Institute of California study showed that Californians' family income at the 10th percentile (inflation adjusted) dropped 14%, from $15,810 in 1969 to $13,600, while those in the 90th percentile increased 58%, from $86,140 in 1969 to $135,850.[10] I believe these large gaps between the rich and the poor contribute to the poor health of individuals and our society. I believe all Americans have the right to decent healthcare and should be treated appropriately regardless of their ability to pay.

Obviously there are multiple factors related to an individual's health and life expectancy. Another study demonstrated how many factors can be significantly and independently associated to a lower life expectancy in the U.S., including the wide income gap among the population, a lack of primary care physicians, the lack of health insurance, less education, higher levels of poverty and smoking.[11] A universal national health program will not solve all of the nation's ills, but it will go a long way towards correcting the current deficiencies in the present system.

Sometimes the system design can offset some of these disparities in income with access to healthcare and insurance. Another study shows how life expectancy at birth correlates to the number of primary care physicians per 10,000 people. New York has a higher density of primary care physicians

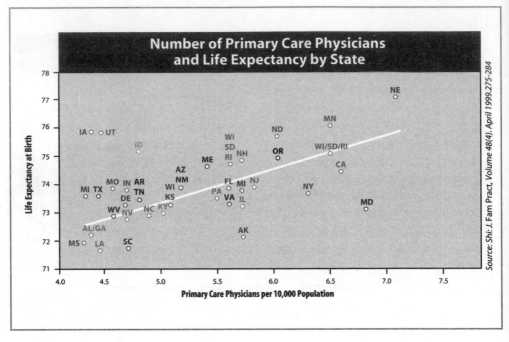

Figure Six

compared to other states and has offset some of the negative effects from this income gap as demonstrated by lower than expected mortality rates. (See Figure Six) Interestingly, Hawaii has among the lowest number of uninsured and also manages to have low mortality rates. (Figure Five on the previous page)

All of the developed countries of the world provide care at significantly lower costs in terms of percentages of gross domestic product compared to the U.S. In 1997, *per capita spending on total healthcare services was $4,090 in the U.S., while the median for the twenty-nine OECD countries was $1,747.*[12]

The 2000 World Health Organization Review of 191 nations ranked the United States as thirty-seventh overall in health system performance, but number one in healthcare costs at 13.7% of GDP or $4,187 per capita in spending. We were also judged to be first in responsiveness to the expectations of the population, including respect for the dignity of individuals, confidentiality of health records, prompt attention in emergencies and widest choice of providers. Despite this "responsiveness," we only ranked twenty-fourth in health or the provision of good health (as measured by life expectancy adjusted for the likelihood of a range of disabilities). The average American has 4.5 years less of good health compared to the citizens of top

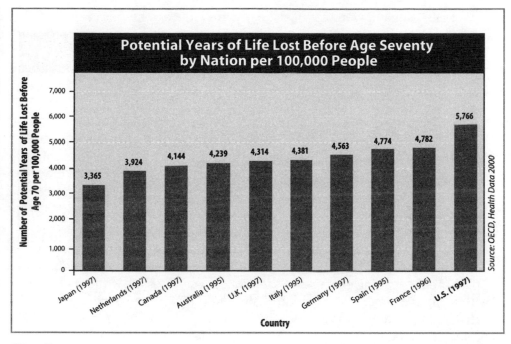

Figure One

ranking Japan. We also rated low, at fifty-fourth, in financial fairness or the fairness of individuals' financial contribution toward their health as measured by the equal distribution of the health costs among households.[13]

The American healthcare lobby and the related industries vilify the systems of other nations. The "excellence" of our system is projected as the standard for the world. Other nations are accused of rationing care and of forcing people into long waiting lines for service. Certainly, they lack the profound market-driven benefits. A closer look at the statistics shows the details of the mediocre performance by the United States. Figure One shows the potential years of life lost before age seventy by nation per 100,000 people. Figure Two on the next page shows higher infant mortality rates compared to other members of the OECD, and Figure Three (see page 117) continues to demonstrate lower life expectancies for men and women.

There are three basic types of healthcare systems we will examine in more detail that have accomplished these results.

Great Britain and Spain are examples of government operated national health services in which doctors and others are mostly salaried. In Britain there are also private hospitals and private insurance for those who wish it.

In a "single-payer" national health insurance system, as in Canada, Denmark, Sweden, and Australia, insurance is publicly administered, and most physicians are in private practice.

Highly regulated, universal multi-payer health insurance systems are in place in countries like Germany, France, The Netherlands, Italy and Japan, which have universal health insurance via sickness funds or similar mechanisms. These funds pay physicians and hospitals uniform rates that are negotiated annually. Also known as an "all-payer" system, participation in the funds is mandatory which makes them essentially funded by the government and taxpayers. Physicians not on hospital or university staffs are in private practice.

National Health Services

These systems are commonly called "socialized medicine." This was the rallying cry by the industry in the initial struggle against universal care in the Truman administration. Great Britain, Finland, Ireland, New Zealand, and Spain are the leading examples. Essentially all services are without charge or with a small charge. The Commonwealth Fund has commissioned surveys of satisfaction with healthcare systems by Louis Harris and Associates. The nations with national health services show generally favorable opinions from

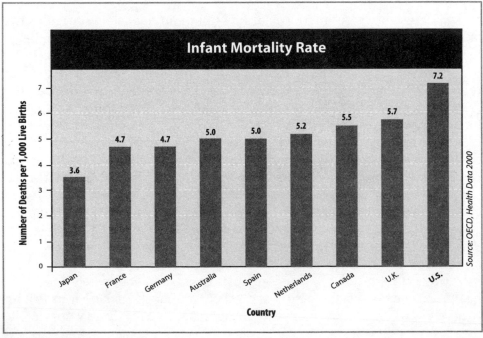

Figure Two

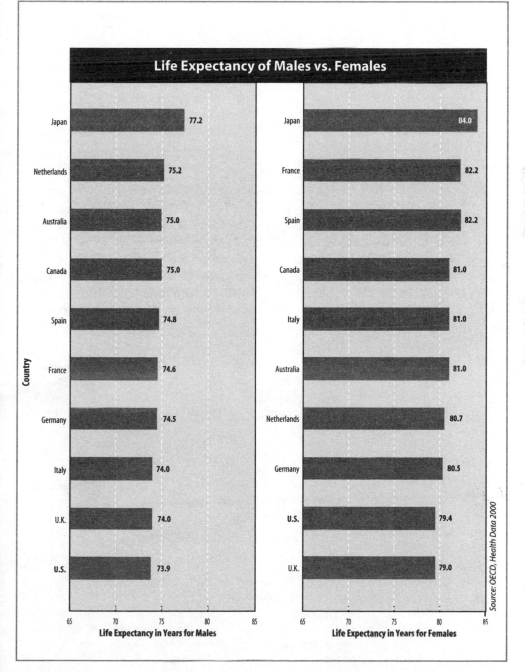

Life Expectancy of Males vs. Females

Life Expectancy in Years for Males

Country	
Japan	77.2
Netherlands	75.2
Australia	75.0
Canada	75.0
Spain	74.8
France	74.6
Germany	74.5
Italy	74.0
U.K.	74.0
U.S.	73.9

Life Expectancy in Years for Females

Country	
Japan	84.0
France	82.2
Spain	82.2
Canada	81.0
Italy	81.0
Australia	81.0
Netherlands	80.7
Germany	80.5
U.S.	79.4
U.K.	79.0

Source: OECD, Health Data 2000

Figure Three

the people they serve. In 1996, a poll in Europe asking for levels of satisfaction by the Harris organization, found people with the following opinions as a percentage of the total:

	Very or fairly satisfied	Neither satisfied nor dissatisfied	Very or fairly dissatisfied
Ireland	49.9	17.4	29.1
Spain	35.6	34.0	28.6
Great Britain	48.1	10.0	40.9

As in all human endeavors, much depends on how well they are managed and funded. Ireland, Spain and Great Britain spend the least of the advanced OECD nations. Almost daily problems with the National Health Service pepper the British newspapers, although some is tabloidism to a degree. In an interview with a longtime member of Parliment, I learned that there is a shortage of doctors and facilities. There are stories of patients dying while waiting for cardiac or other emergency surgery.[14] The statistics show that the British system is under-funded relative to the other wealthy OECD nations. Recently, funding for the system and doctors has been increased. Regardless of their under-funding, the ultimate analysis demonstrates the U.K. has lower infant mortality and lower premature deaths rates compared to the U.S.[15] See Figures One and Two, on pages 115 and 116.

The Spanish Constitution, adopted after the collapse of the Franco regime, cites healthcare as a basic human right. The system is funded from a payroll tax with 75% paid by the employer and 25% by the employee. This is paid to the Instituto Nacional de Salute, the National Institute of Health. The majority of care is provided through clinics and hospitals where doctors are salaried. Medical education is free to qualified students. The ratings by the patients are not high. I suspect one issue may be that the clinic idea does not provide for people to have their own doctors. However, overall health outcomes are uniformly better than in the United States.

The Single-Payer National Health Insurance Systems

If all the people in this country were on Medicare, we would have a single-payer system. Medicare collects a tax and then pays the bills of doctors, hospitals, nursing homes and other caregivers. The Centers for Medicare and Medicaid Services, previously named the Healthcare Finance Administration (HCFA), administers Medicare with an overhead cost of about 2.0%.[16] Significant additional administrative costs are thrust upon the private insurers, providers and patients.

In a single-payer system, most of the hospitals are community owned or, in some cases, regionally owned. Doctors on staff are frequently salaried; most other doctors are in private practice. The funds are administered regionally or locally. Nations using this concept have some variations:

CANADA: The program, also called "medicare," is funded from general tax revenues and administered by the Provinces. They use a small "m" to demonstrate the lack of administrative oversight and cost. Unlike the current U.S. Medicare program which has over 100,000 pages of rules and related documents, the original draft of the Canadian Healthcare Act was approximately ten pages in length. Doctors in private practice accept fee-for-service rates set in negotiation with the provinces and also have fees for their private patients. Most Canadians have supplemental insurance for dental work, prescriptions, rehabilitation and nursing care. Of the total expenditure, 72% is from the national system which covers everyone. Insurance companies pay 20% and patients pay 8% out-of-pocket. This is in contrast to over 17% out-of-pocket costs for the average American.[17]

In a recent international survey of physicians from five nations, 61% of the American doctors reported U.S. patients often have difficulty affording their out-of-pocket costs, significantly higher than Canadian, British and Australian doctors' reports. Over one half of the U.S. doctors were very concerned that patients will not be able to afford the care they need, again significantly greater than the other nations. Significant differences also were found in comparison to Canadian physicians. U.S. doctors reported more patients getting sicker because they are unable to get the care they need and often do not receive preventive care.[18]

I hear Americans blast the Canadian system for many reasons, including the phenomenon labeled "brain drain." This implies smart people will be less likely to enter the medical profession or may leave the profession after training, because of their nation's health system. Americans, as well as Canadians, need to realize the truth about both nations' systems.

Since 1992, Canadian physicians moving abroad ranged from a high of 777 in 1994 to a low of 569 in 1998 with 585 in 1999 or 1.0% of their total physician workforce. Physicians returning to Canada from abroad and resuming active status ranged from a low of 218 in 1996 to a high of 343 in 1999. The "net loss" from moving out of Canada was 242 in 1999 or 0.42% of total physicians. And of those moving abroad in 1999, only 31% were general or family practitioners and 8% were leaving the country after more than thirty years of practice in Canada.[19] I suspect many of these doctors were retiring to warmer climates. In the year 2000, first-year allopathic medical students were 5.55 per 100,000 population in Canada, a 12% increase from 1997, while the U.S.

had 6.00 first year students per 100,000 population in 1998, a 1.9% decrease from 1993.[20] There are twice as many medical school applicants per place in Canada than in the U.S. Both countries rely on a significant international physician workforce with approximately one out of every four doctors being trained abroad.[21]

This is not to say there is not a "brain drain" problem in Canada, but the United States may be facing an even greater one. According to one survey, 38% of our physicians who are fifty years of age and older plan to retire in the next three years and another 10% plan non-direct patient care employment in that same time frame.[22] According to these figures, I estimate the U.S. may lose 40,000 physicians per year over the next three years, or 5.1% per year of all U.S. physicians. A more recent survey of 2,300 physicians in California shows that 43% of them plan to leave medical practice in California over the next three years.[23] Of all Canadian physicians, only 3.5% retire, die, emigrate or leave practice per year.[24] I think we may have a greater "brain drain" problem in the states.

The United States does have more doctors than Canada, with 2.7 physicians per 1,000 people compared to 2.1 per 1,000. Other nations show rates with France at 3.0, Germany at 3.5, Great Britain at 1.7 and Japan at 1.9 per 1,000.[25] Rural, non-metropolitan areas in the U.S., comprising 24% of the entire population (roughly twice the population size of Canada), face total physician ratios of 1.2 per 1,000. To offset this physician shortage, we employ 23.5% more nurse practitioners in rural versus urban communities.[26] Some may argue this is also a "brain drain" phenomenon. And even more disturbing for rural Americans, they face lower household incomes and higher poverty rates. Rural providers and hospitals are expected to treat the elderly at 82% of the rate of urban Medicare reimbursement.[27] No wonder rural Americans face more functional disability and poor health.

However, using the U.S. definition of a primary care physician (PCP), the U.S. has fewer PCP, 1.0 per 1000, compared to Canada, 1.3 per 1,000. America does have twice the number of specialists.[28] In 1997, Canadian doctors averaged approximately $120,000 (in U.S. dollars) in annual income, while our doctors averaged $165,000.[29] Our physicians work longer hours, averaging five hours more per week. Considering our failure to provide decent healthcare to all people from the beginning of their lives, we may need U.S. doctors working longer hours and more specialists to care for the higher incidences of serious illness that results.

DENMARK: The health system is funded by a progressive income tax. The hospitals are run by the counties or by the large city of Copenhagen. The doctors on staff are salaried according to union negotiations. All others are in private practice. The specialists receive fees; the general practitioners a capitation and a fee for service. Danes are encouraged to select a primary care physician who makes referrals to specialists.

SWEDEN: The system, which covers everyone, is primarily funded by a progressive income tax and is operated by county councils. These councils own the hospitals and employ physicians for the staff, a majority of general practices and outpatient facilities. Some physicians are in private practice and receive fee-for-service payments. There are small payments from individuals for services, hospitalization and prescriptions. The maximum an individual pays is under $300 per year, about a third of the cost of a one-day stay in a U.S. hospital. The cost of medical school education is covered for Swedish students accepted into graduate school.

In the Louis Harris surveys by the OECD the single-payer nations do well:

	Very or fairly satisfied	Neither satisfied or dissatisfied	Very or fairly dissatisfied
Denmark	90.0	3.8	5.7
Finland	86.4	7.0	6.0
Luxumberg	71.1	16.1	8.9
Sweden	67.3	16.7	14.2

The Universal Multi-payer Insurance Systems

There are subtle differences between the universal care multi-payer and single-payer systems. In universal care multi-payer systems, hospitals are mostly community owned, but can be privately owned, and in rare instances are for-profit. Physicians on staff are salaried; the others are in private practice receiving set fees negotiated with the payers. These are most commonly called "sickness funds" into which funds are paid. They are usually managed by insurance companies or are insurance companies themselves. Participation is mandatory and extra insurance is available. Staff members of Olin-Frederick interviewed doctors in Germany to learn more about their health system and to hear directly from providers about the system's performance.

GERMANY: All Germans are required to buy into what is called statutory insurance if they have incomes of less than a certain amount, currently 6,000 Deutsche Marks (DM) per month. Those with higher incomes can opt out of the system in favor of private insurance, but they must buy it. This requires 12 to 15% of wages and salaries to be placed into a variety of sickness funds. These percentages can change and the high-income level can change. There is a minimum of 600 to 800 DM every three months that students pay. Private insurance is less expensive than the statutory insurance because the latter must take everyone. Six thousand DM at a realistic exchange rate is about 3,500 U.S. dollars

Private insurance companies take only healthy people and investigate health backgrounds of potential clients before accepting them. The premiums vary for private insurance. Most Germans who can take private insurance generally stay with the statutory program. Alcohol and drug addiction are covered by the statutory program but not by private insurance unless the addiction was known prior to the insurance being purchased.

Germany has more doctors than any other major OECD nation. They are well paid, second only to the United States. Medical education is free to those who win places in the medical schools. The same is true for nursing. Doctors on hospital staffs are salaried. The others, over half of which are specialists, work in private practice and are paid on a fee-for-service basis. While it is unofficial, the interviewed doctors defined the "WANZ principle," a German acronym for providers only doing what is economical, satisfactory, necessary, and pragmatic (Wirtschaftlich-Ausreichend-Notwendig-Zweckmaessing). Doctors are not necessarily asked to do their very best, only that which is satisfactory. This principle obviously is not the ideal building block for a sound healthcare system or professional code of ethics.

The German doctors also complain about excessive bureaucracy. Numerous patient tests and procedures require approval from the insurance companies, similar to the United States. Unlike America, all Germans have an insurance card that is swiped at the doctor's office or hospital to start the payment process. The doctors do what they think is satisfactory within the confines of their system. Despite the WANZ principal Germany's health record is still better than the U.S., but is below the European averages.[30]

FRANCE: They also have a multi-payer system in this country with a national headquarter and regional networks. Sickness funds are supported by payroll deductions and taxes on the employers for each employee. Other professionals or the self-employed pay into these funds based on their income. The government also subsidizes the sickness funds from general revenues. The system is under the French Social Security (Securite Social) and The Ministry of Health. There is a National Office of Sickness Insurance (Caisse National d'Assurances Maladie) with regional and local offices. Everyone is covered for basic insurance and may choose additional options.

In contrast to the U.S., explicit principles underlie the French health system. One is the shared perception that government has the prime responsibility to protect all citizens and permanent residents against having to pay large out-of-pocket costs for healthcare. A second is intergenerational solidarity which acknowledges that the younger, working generation will subsidize the older generation. A third principle is inter-group cross-subsidization. Additional key principles, incorporated in the 1979 Code of Ethics, include free choice of physician and freedom for physicians to treat patients as they see fit. Physicians can establish ambulatory practice wherever they choose.[31]

One-third of the doctors arc employed by public hospitals.[32] There are private hospitals, a few of which are for-profit. All other doctors are in private practice and receive agreed on fees for service. There are no limits on the service, and in 1978 when the system was legislatively finalized, a law was passed making the decisions of the doctors final. French doctors have no insurance reviewers, no HMO administrators, and no lawyers interfering with their efforts to treat and cure their patients. Medical and nursing school education costs are paid by the government.

The French also complain about the bureaucracy. The method of payment is partially from the patient, who then receives reimbursement from the insurance fund. Thus, the fund deals not with only practitioners but also with the citizens in France who will not tolerate delays in payments.

JAPAN: The laws concerning the healthcare system were passed in 1958 and the system fully implemented in 1962. While Japan again has multiple funds, as payers it is organized differently. There is an Employees Health Insurance System, financed by payroll withdrawals of 8%, half from the employer. The National Health Insurance System covers the self-employed and pensioners and their dependents. The premiums are set according to income and assets. Both are divided into functional units serving particular social or economic groups like farmers, professionals, and various industries to simplify administration. Local governments act as insurers.

Most hospitals and clinics are privately owned but for-profit hospitals are prohibited. Doctors not on staff are in private practice receiving established fees for service. They also have another perk. They sell pharmaceuticals to their patients. Any estimates of the income of Japanese physicians must be adjusted by additional income from prescription sales.

ITALY: Italians are universally covered by a health system called the Servizio Sanitario Nazionale (SSN). The system is the same for young and old, rich and poor. Mental illness and drug addiction treatments are covered.

Some patients may pay out-of-pocket and opt out of the public system due to "waiting lines," and thus are paying for private healthcare. Physicians, general practitioners and specialists are paid by the SSN. However, some people wish to choose their specialist or receive specialty care sooner, preferring to pay more out-of-pocket for better access.

Most hospitals are public unless located in under-serviced areas. Patients under the public system do not have to pay for hospitalizations or physician services. Waiting lines for emergency care are rare, and the access to high-tech medical services is "good". Bureaucracy is also a common complaint of their system. Overall average out-of pocket costs are high, the second highest in the world, probably due to their private care option.

Italians rarely go outside of Italy to obtain health services. They have a strong medical establishment, including R&D, which has contributed many new medicines and advanced technologies.

The OECD survey findings from 1997 on the multiple payers is:

	Very or fairly Satisfied%	Neither satisfied nor dissatisfied%	Very or fairly dissatisfied%
Austria	63.3	27.6	4.7
France	65.1	18.7	14.6
Germany	66.0	2.4	10.9
Netherlands	67.3	8.8	17.4

An earlier study also demonstrated various nations' satisfaction in relationship to the cost of their healthcare systems, as shown in Figure Seven. I believe the Italians probably dislike their system primarily because of their high out-of-pocket costs while the Spanish and British people obviously underfund their system. In the United States, we fail to provide universal coverage and face the highest costs overall in the world. Those nations providing universal coverage, adequate funding and lower out-of-pocket costs seem to have the highest patient satisfaction.

A CBS News poll of Americans asked for opinions on whether minor changes were needed, whether or not fundamental changes were needed, or if the system needed to be rebuilt. One out of four indicated that the system should be totally rebuilt and over 60% said fundamental changes are needed in the U.S.[33] Again, this suggests substantial dissatisfaction. A key question now is which nations should be compared to the United States? I have chosen the next nine largest democratic, industrialized nations of the OECD: Japan, Germany, France, Great Britain (U.K.), Italy, Canada, Spain, Australia, and The Netherlands.

Figures One, Two and Three, see pages 115, 116 and 117, confirm that the United States continues to present poorly in the overall health of its people. I believe "unsatisfactory" is a better term. Many people don't like the healthcare system. A substantial reason for this disenchantment has a great deal to do with money. Those who want to preserve their access to the cash flow deny the access of all Americans to healthcare that is provided in every other nation. Whichever of the market-driven motives they propound, the usual cry is that universal care will cost too much and ruin our great system.

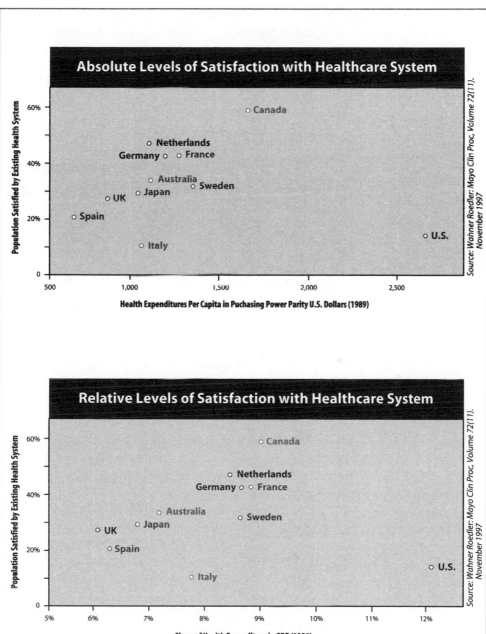

Source: Wahner Roedler: Mayo Clin Proc, Volume 72(11). November 1997

Figure Seven

The Universal Declaration of Human Rights by the United Nations called for universal healthcare. This declaration was adopted by the General Assembly of the United Nations on December 10, 1948.[34] Since that time every country has adopted a universal health program for their nation except the United States. South Africa implemented a national health program in 1996 and established healthcare as a human right in their constitution only after the destruction of apartheid.

Article twenty-five of The Universal Declaration of Human Rights states:

1. *Everyone has the right to a standard of living adequate for the health and well being of himself and of his family.* This includes food, clothing, housing, medical care, necessary social services, and the right to security. This right is extended in the event of unemployment, sickness, disability, widowhood, old age or other lack of livelihood in circumstances beyond his control.

2. Motherhood and childhood are entitled to special care and assistance. All children, whether born in or out of wedlock, shall enjoy the same social protection.

When I examined the comparison nations' health costs as a percentage of GDP and the relationship to public financing, private financing, or out-of-pocket costs, there was a surprise for Americans who believe their healthcare lobby. Those nations that fund a larger percentage of their health services under a *publicly* funded system, spend less money overall for healthcare as a percentage of GDP. See Figure Eight. Those nations that fund a larger percentage of their health services under a *privately* funded system and private insurance spend more overall for healthcare as a percentage of GDP. See Figure Nine.[35] These international comparisons and findings are the exact opposite of the current "dogma" in U.S. politics today.

When I examined these international comparisons, out-of-pocket costs had no correlation, positively or negatively, to total healthcare costs as a percent of GDP. However, placing more out-of-pocket costs on patients can cause more serious illness and higher mortality rates. Recent studies have shown how dangerous rising out-of-pocket costs can be for the poor or sick. When Canadian patients were forced to pay more out-of-pocket for prescriptions, their emergency room visits and adverse outcomes increased.[36] An American study showed a 25% increase in mortality rates for the elderly sick and poor when they faced higher out-of-pocket costs.[37] No wealthy democratic nation will save any money overall by placing more costs onto sick or poor patients. The current U.S. policy of placing higher costs onto the patients through higher deductibles, co-pays and less insurance coverage will harm the very patients the system is designed to serve. The people and leaders of the United States must understand that there are two internationally proven

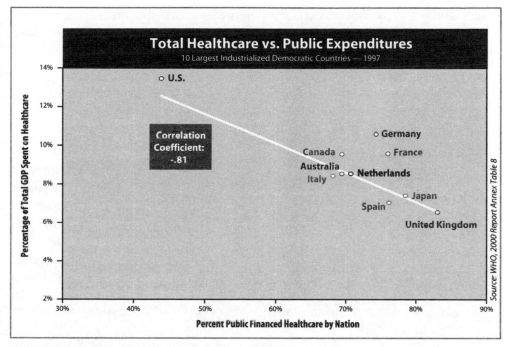

Figure Eight

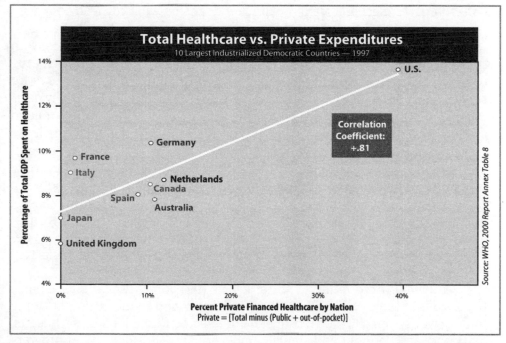

Figure Nine

and effective techniques to control healthcare costs: universal coverage and public financing.[38] This may be a shocking truth for some Americans, but I suspect many in leadership positions already know these facts.

In a single-payer system with simplified financing, all would share the cost of universal coverage and also share the benefits, while more fairly distributing the cost of universal coverage for everyone. Everyone would be covered continuously.

The health industry lobby and associated special interest groups in this country will oppose a single-payer, comprehensive, universal system. The for-profit healthcare industries gain from the current sick system. The doctors are the highest paid in the world. The drug companies are the most profitable major industry in the country. The for-profit insurance companies and HMOs return profits to their shareholders and exploit the cash flow. The lawyers benefit from the largest number of malpractice cases and settlements in the world, as well as from the mountains of legal contracts and disputes. Elected officials and political parties cash in on the multiple campaign donors who fund their re-election campaigns. The hospital industry has the highest costs and largest administrative staffs in the world. For some there are advantages!

Conventional wisdom in the U.S. believes the market will correct high costs through market forces of supply and demand. Many disagree and believe market mechanisms in healthcare financing will only lead to advantages for certain groups. They explain how privately funded healthcare systems, compared to publicly funded systems, have higher overall costs, with these higher revnues and incomes passed on to the providers, doctors, drug companies, private insurance companies and others. Private payments for services also distribute system costs according to use, thus potentially costing the healthy and wealthy people less compared to a publicly funded system. And the remaining wealthy patients, can purchase higher quality or better access to healthcare without having to support a similar standard of care for the less fortunate members of society. One author wrote, "Thus there is, and always has been, a natural alliance of economic interest between service providers and upper-income citizens to support shifting health financing from public to private sources."[39] In America, the world's most expensive health system, the lack of a national health program and single-payer public funding leads to higher costs for everyone and unsatisfactory health outcomes.

A General Accounting Office study in 1991 forecast that single-payer healthcare in the U.S. would drastically simplify and reduce the cost of the multi-payer system.[40] Three recent state studies performed in Massachusetts, Maryland, and Vermont had similar conclusions.[41, 42] A single-payer program in the U.S. would not increase the percentage of GDP spent on healthcare, currently 13.9% in 1999.

Healthcare Inflation

Some claim the high cost of healthcare arose as a result of governmental insurance programs such as Medicare and Medicaid in the 1960s. The facts show that Medicare's inflation and growth have been significantly less over the past three decades compared to private health insurance in the United States. From 1969 to 1998, Medicare spending increased by 1,562%, while private insurers' spending rose by 2,165%, 40% more than Medicare.[43] In the year 2000, Medicare spending actually went down one percent, while private insurance continues to track substantially above inflation with an average increase of 11% in 2000, and 8.1% in 1999.[44] Medicare provides the bulk of services to the oldest and sickest members of our society. For instance, Medicare patients account for 83% of all deaths in this country, as would be expected in nearly 100% coverage of seniors. In addition, Medicare automatically covers all patients on hemodialysis, and they are some of the sickest patients I have ever known. Additional research again shows how public financing of healthcare more likely controls inflation. See Figure Ten. According to this researcher, the less medical services were publically

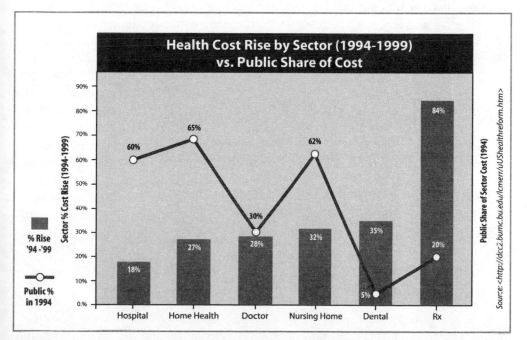

Figure Ten

funded, the higher the inflation rate in the 1990s. This appears especially true for dental and prescription services, two areas where tens of millions of Americans lack coverage.[45] Preventing patients from receiving necessary medical services does not control inflation either.

Healthcare inflation is rising more in the U.S. compared to the other wealthy OECD nations. Countries with universal health insurance and publicly funded healthcare programs fared better with less inflation during the past twenty to thirty years.[46] Private health insurance has been unable to control healthcare inflation in America and around the world. When will the world, especially America, realize this fact?

There have been instances of severe inflation in America. Between 1979 and 1980 the Consumer Price Index (CPI) rose 13.5%, driven by energy price increases. The price levels of the items making up the CPI increased 2.2% from 1998 to 1999. This is also inflation but to a lesser degree; Americans seem to tolerate low levels of inflation.[47]

In narrowly defined markets a few competitors can monitor each other. Sometimes, one of them with a major cost cutting or product improvement technology, will attack the others. Often joint price increases result. One raises the price and the others follow. In business the quickest way to increase profits is raising the price and getting customers to pay it.

I mentioned before that the demand for healthcare is "inelastic." This means it is something that people have to buy in some quantity in order to survive. Medical care is a necessity which can be exploited by those business owners, shareholders, or executives who do not identify their interests with social consciousness.

In the case of water, electric power, and transportation, governments intervene and regulate the prices and plan the availability. When governments do not regulate, shortages and high prices, like those that beset California in early 2001, occur. The real and fundamental reason was the United States had no energy policy, as the previous administrations found themselves caught between the need for energy and environmental protection.

The United States also has no national healthcare policy. Every other industrialized nation has one based on the United Nations Declaration of 1948. Without a national policy things get out of hand. The Bureau of Labor Statistics supplies some further information.[48]

Index of Healthcare Prices in the United States (%)

Consumer Price Index (CPI) base years of 1982-1984 = 100%

	CPI%	Total healthcare	Physicians	Hospitals and supplies	Pharmaceuticals
1980	82.4	74.8	76.5	69.2	72.5
1985	107.6	133.5	113.3	116.1	120.1
1990	130.7	162.8	160.8	178.0	181.7
1995	152.4	220.5	208.8	257.8	235.0
1999	166.6	250.6	236.0	299.5	273.4

Doctors have joined the elite of the nation by increasing their incomes faster than the rate of inflation, as rendered by the CPI. They have also experienced the higher costs of dealing with multiple insurers. The margin of difference is that physicians' collections rose at a rate 106% faster than the CPI and more than doubled in twenty years. Pharmaceuticals increased 2.8 times and hospital billings more than tripled at 3.3 times the prices of 1980. There could be many reasons for this increase, but one surely is the lack of national planning and policy. Some states do well and have responded to the needs with their own policies. Others have not or simply lack the resources.

The solution is to forge a health policy that, among other things, prevents such increases beyond the stream of inflation. The comparison nations have such policies which entail negotiating fees and charges and have much lower hospital costs. Many of the nations pay for the medical education of doctors and dentists so that young people do not come out of their training owing six figures for education loans. The funds to pay for the education debts are also after-tax dollars. These large debts press U.S. doctors and dentists to seek high incomes in their early professional years. Doctors in the comparison nations do not face these severe economic "start-up" costs.

The comparison nations have healthcare inflation but it is still significantly less than in the U.S. From 1998 to 1999 when U.S. prices increased 3.5%, the comparison reporting nations averaged 1.6%.[49] A national healthcare program must provide accessible, quality care to every citizen and at the same time restrain the exploitation of the inelastic market by those who would exploit the market. Regrettably, the fact that the two actions go together is the reason for the extreme resistance by the healthcare industry to having such a national policy. More regrettable, is the fact that so many Americans have suffered unnecessary illness, early disability and early death waiting for such a policy to be instituted. So where does all the money for healthcare go in America?

8: THE COSTS

"In the circle of life you should not take more than you give."

Elton John

Some cannot find the heart or the mindset to support comprehensive quality healthcare for all people in this nation despite the obvious basic human need. They must respond, however, to an economic analysis proving why the United States must enact a national healthcare program. In this chapter I will show the total costs and excesses of American healthcare using 1998 as the reference year, the last for which comprehensive data is available. This will demonstrate the enormous excessive costs and illnesses Americans suffer under our sick system. I will further prove through four different analyses that Americans spend approximately $160 billion in excess costs caring for patients who are sick, who would not have been sick had they lived in the comparison nations with universal health systems.

Whenever possible, the industry and its lobbies avoid any discussion of the costs paid by the American people for healthcare. Many in government and healthcare are aware of the statistics, but few call attention to the fact that our costs are far greater than in other OECD nations. The comparison most often used is the amount of healthcare expense as a percentage of a nation's Gross Domestic Product (GDP). The GDP data for 1998 for the ten largest industrialized democratic OECD countries is in Figures Eleven and Twelve. The U.S. is indeed the economic colossus, generating nearly one-fifth of the world's total GDP despite only having 5% of the world's population. A single percentage point of the American GDP was $83 billion in 1998.[1]

Healthcare costs in the United States are also an economic colossus amounting to 58% more than the weighted average of the comparison nations, the nine largest industrialized democracies in the OECD after the U.S. In 1998 Americans spent 13.6% of GDP on healthcare, or $4,178 per capita. The total was $1,149.1 billion. The weighted average of the comparison nations

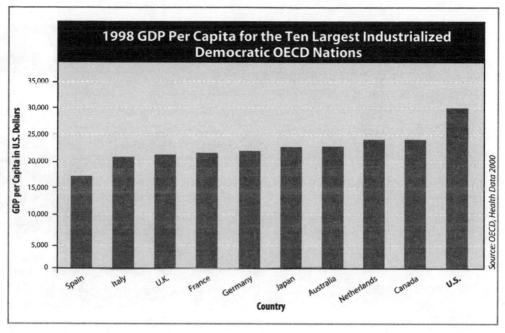

Figure Eleven

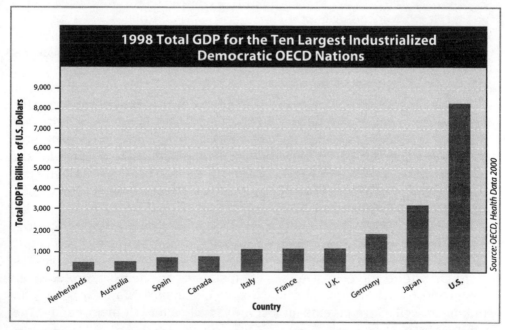

Figure Twelve

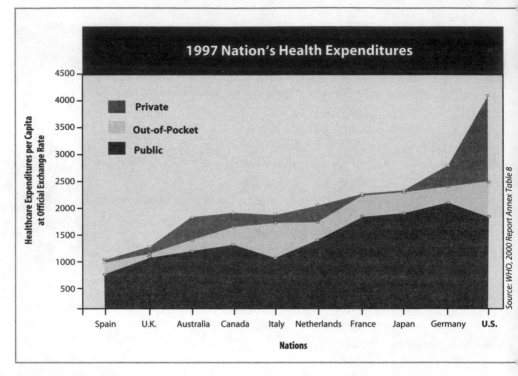

Figure Thirteen

was 8.47% of GDP or $1,905 per capita.[2] This is calculated in U.S. dollars by purchasing power parity, which adjusts the currency market exchange rate to selected prices in other nations.

The differential of greater expenditure on healthcare between the U.S. and the comparison nations was 5.14% of GDP. This is huge, totaling $428 billion. This is more than the total GDP of Switzerland and Austria combined. It was 1.4 times the U.S. defense budget. Compared to the average for the comparison nations, we spent $2,273 more per capita or $5,908 more per household for healthcare.[3] See Figure Thirteen. (The estimated U.S. population was 270.3 million living in 102,538,000 households in 1998)

Make no mistake as to who pays. Many Americans never think about paying a medical bill. They pay their insurance company to let them worry about it. Competently managed companies who want the best people working for them offer comprehensive medical insurance so their employees never have to worry about medical costs. Medical insurance is a high priority for unions as well. Governments almost universally offer full medical coverage for their employees.

Local, real estate, sales and income taxes; state sales, excise, income and business taxes; and federal income, excise and business taxes, the Medicare tax, and alcohol and tobacco taxes are used to fund the programs at all levels. The federal role is Medicare and Medicaid supplements; the states contribute to Medicaid and operate state hospitals and facilities; local jurisdictions supplement the community hospitals and a multitude of health activities. Clinics and hospitals inflate their bills to get the funds they need to keep open and provide full services. Doctors do the same. Every American pays something; but collectively individuals pay it all from their income.

When challenged, the American healthcare industry and its combined lobbies shrug off the massive differential in cost as what is required for a market-driven or "the best" healthcare system. As has been shown, American results are far from the best. Americans are not healthier than the citizens of the comparison nations. Americans are not as healthy. The question is: what are we paying for that costs each household so much more than families in other nations? The differential in cost contains eight apparent factors, which could account for the astronomic excess. They are:

- Excesses in pharmaceutical marketing.
- Higher prices for the same pharmaceuticals sold worldwide.
- Higher physician incomes.
- Higher costs of multiple insurance companies and HMOs.
- Excess administrative costs as a result of the multi-payer structure.
- Better and more diagnostic, therapeutic and surgical equipment.
- Defensive medicine to protect practitioners against plaintiff lawyers.
- Larger per capita expenditures on research.

There is a ninth variable causing the differential which may be the most significant. It is that we have a greater number of sick people in the United States as opposed to the comparison nations, and the rest of the industrialized OECD, who would not have been ill if they had been treated in a universal healthcare system. According to a 2001 *Health Affairs* report, 5.4 million Americans consume 38% of the healthcare costs in the United States.[4] They are the seriously ill. I believe it is evident and I will further show that one quarter of these patients' illnesses would have been prevented with a decent universal health system. Some may think 1.35 million people doesn't sound like many. In this book I have told the stories of those in my practice. There is no question that there are numerous Americans who are sick who would not be if they lived in Europe, Australia, Canada, or Japan, where they would have had accessible primary and preventive care.

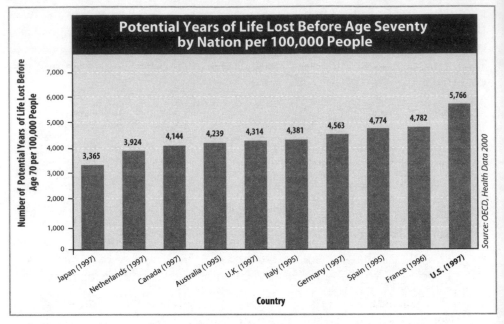

Figure One

For nearly two generations most of the comparison nations have provided basic healthcare to everyone. As a result these nations have fewer sick people for whom to care. The average American becomes disabled sooner, spends a greater portion of his life disabled and is more likely to die a premature death. See Figure One. Americans may be suffering premature death and years of life lost far greater than the average of the comparison nations—a number that is over twenty times the life years lost by the horrendous terrorist attack on the World Trade Center and the Pentagon. In the U.S. a greater percentage of uninsured and underinsured citizens have become ill, resulting in larger rates of illness and higher costs compared to the weighted averages of the comparison nations. Americans pay for the care of over three million citizens, counting the less seriously ill, who would not be sick if they had access to universal care from the beginning. Prevention can be significantly less expensive than cures and treatments of many diseases.

THE DIFFERENTIAL AND THE GAP

In theory, Americans are evidently willing to pay more for better care, spending more for pharmaceuticals, providers, well-equipped facilities and research. But the differential with the comparison nations is very large at 5.1% of GDP or $428 billion. The reality is the American people are paying an enormous amount of money annually for the citizens who are sick because they did not have access to primary and preventive care. I will show that the cost in 1998 was approximately $160 billion. There is ample evidence of this. The breakdown of the American healthcare expense for 1998 and the average cost to each of the 102,538,000 households was:[5]

ITEM	Total (Billions)	Average/ Household
Pharmaceuticals, OTC, vitamins	$121.9	$1,189
Doctors office visits and treatments	$229.5	$2,238
Hospital treatment	$382.8	$3,733
Dental care	$53.8	$525
Other professional services	$66.6	$650
Nursing home care	$87.8	$856
Home care	$29.3	$286
Vision products and other durables	$15.5	$151
Other health services	$32.1	$313
Sub Total	**$1,019.3**	**$9,941**
Net cost of insurance and administration	$57.7	$563
Public health activities	$36.6	$357
Total expenses	**$1,113.6**	**$10,860**
Publicly funded medical research	$19.9	$194
Medical facilities construction	$15.5	$152
Total with research and construction	**$1,149.0**	**$11,206**

The total of U.S. health expenditures as measured by the OECD, probably leaves out construction and related costs and shows a total for the U.S. of $1,129.2 billion or $11,012 per household. The estimated average total expenditures for healthcare in the comparison nations was $4,951 per household.[6] The analysis of the differential of $428 billion between the U.S. and the comparison nations is revealing.

The Cost of Pharmaceuticals

In 1998 the sales of prescription drugs in the U.S. were about $91 billion.[7] See Figure Fourteen on page 138. Of this revenue, 22% was used for marketing expense.[8] In Britain an agreement between the National Health Service and the pharmaceutical industry allows 9% of revenue to be used for marketing.[9] And remember the U.S. is the only nation in the world to allow direct-to-consumer advertising for prescription drugs. If we used a figure of 10% marketing costs to meet the needs of patients and providers for the U.S. pharmaceutical industry, then 12% would be an overage, or approximately $10.9 billion in excess expense.

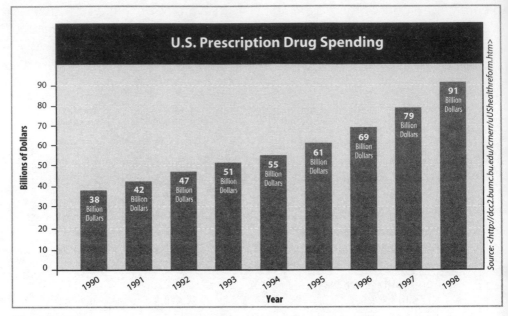

Figure Fourteen

Compared to the norm for other American industries, the pharmaceutical manufacturers have high selling, general and administrative expenses.[10] Harsh critics may say that the excess cost of $4 billion in expenses, other than marketing and research, and that the after tax profits of over 18% of revenue are too high. The industry, however, may have a greater need for highly trained professionals and are producing results of potential great benefit. The industry is also the most profitable in America, but it takes unusual risks and therefore high profits may be justified. This is particularly true if a good portion of the profits are used to fund new projects or capital expansion. If all patients could afford and had equal access to their products, I would not object to the industry's high profits.

There is also a question of the prices charged. Figure Four shows a comparison researched by the Canadian Patented Medicine Price Review Board. This is a government commission, that watches the prices of drugs around the world. It is clear that the patented ones are more expensive in the United States. However, not all pharmaceuticals are patented. Many patents have run their course on commonly prescribed drugs. In 2001 it is estimated that Americans will spend $484 per person for prescription drugs, which is $73 or 20% more than the next highest country, France. The OECD indicates that in 1998, however, the difference between the U.S. and French payments was only 11%, $335 versus $297and that the payments in Japan the year before were $276. Of the other comparison nations reporting, Great Britain

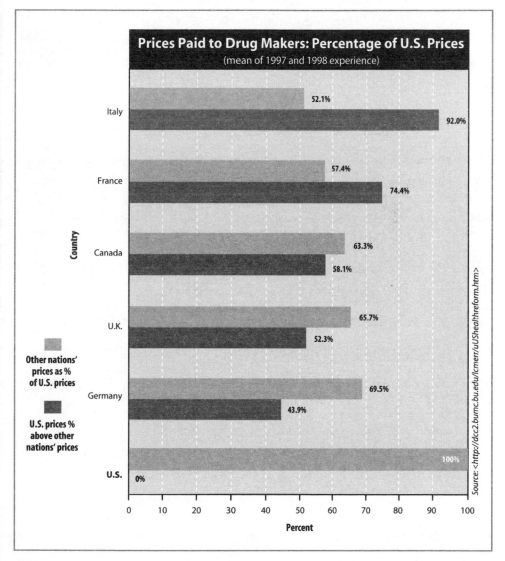

Figure Four

and Australia, show a much lower per capita use in 1997 of $157 and $153 per capita.[11] Because these nations have a largely government-operated system the meaning of the data is not certain.

A macro analysis of the pharmaceutical industry presented in the reference notes indicates that 20% is the most the overall higher margins could be for sales in the United States. In my judgment, a reasonable estimate is that U.S. patients paid 15% more for their prescriptions in 1998, contributing $13.7 billion in excess American expenditure versus the comparison nations.[12] This is $133 per household. The pharmaceutical portion of the differential of higher American healthcare costs is estimated to be $24.6 billion, or $240 per household.

Physicians' Income

Taxable and nontaxable physicians' collections in 1998 were $229 billion according to the Healthcare Financing Administration (HCFA).[13] The American Medical Association, through a survey, regularly measures physicians' income and expenses. Their calculations of specialists showed their income to be 46.6% of total collections.[14] This is the physicians' salaries or their share of practice profits. The balance covers nursing, administrative, office and equipment costs. The total income of physicians in the United States is estimated by using the AMA ratio and the Census' revenue figures at $106.7 billion. U.S. physicians, who must finance their own education and practice entry, are paid about double the incomes of the physicians in the comparison nations. See the reference for details.[15] This means that for the higher salaries or income of doctors, Americans pay $53.4 billion more in total or $529 more per household than citizens of the comparison nations.

The Cost of Insurance and the HMOs

In 1998, $375 billion was paid as private insurance premiums in the U.S., including HMOs.[16] Of this amount, $137.1 billion went to for-profit insurance companies, which in turn paid $113.8 billion in benefits with an underwriting margin of $23.3 billion or 17%.[17] The balance, $237.9 billion, was paid into not-for-profit insurance companies, which took an underwriting margin of a reported 11.4% or $29.1 billion.[18] Thus the total underwriting cost of the insurance in 1998 was $52.4 billion. There are further reported costs for insurance and administration of $5.3 billion.[19] The important figure is the amount to which American underwriting expense exceeds that of the comparison nations and is part of the higher American costs. The OECD offers the following table of national expenditure for insurance and administration as a percentage of GDP:[20]

	1990	1991	1992	1993	1994	1995	1996	1997	1998	1999
Canada	0.2	0.2	0.2	0.2	0.2	0.2	0.2	0.2	0.2	0.2
France	0.1	0.1	0.1	0.1	0.2	0.2	0.2	0.2	0.2	0.2
Germany	0.5	0.5	0.5	0.6	0.6	0.6	0.6	0.7	0.7	0.7
Netherlands	0.4	0.4	0.4	0.4	0.4	0.4	0.4	0.4	0.4	0.4
Switzerland	0.5	0.5	0.5	0.5	0.5	0.5	0.5	0.5	0.6	0.5
USA	0.6	0.7	0.7	0.7	0.8	0.8	0.8	0.7	0.6	0.7

All of the single-payer nations, except Canada and Britain, rely on a form of public insurance that is operated by the private insurance companies with government contributions. In Germany there are multiple insurance companies. Germany has the highest total expenditure on healthcare of the comparison nations in terms of the percentage of GDP at 10.6%.[21] France also uses insurance channels in healthcare, but at a much lower cost than Germany. In the European countries, with reduced involvement by insurance companies, the cost in percent of GDP is lower. For purposes of establishing a difference between the U.S. and the comparison nations, there is an anomaly regarding Germany. The following table from the OECD shows the total and per capita insurance underwriting and administrative costs in 1998 in U.S. dollars at purchasing power parity. These expenses *do not* include the administrative cost to doctors and hospitals.

Per Capita Insurance and Underwriting Costs (OECD 2000)

	Total ($ millions)	$ Per Capita
Australia	$ 1,092	$ 58
Canada	1,544	51
France	2,710	37
Germany	12,293	150
Netherlands	1,231	78
United States	57,743	214

The German policy, we know, is flawed in somewhat the same way as the American. There are multiple payers. The other comparison nations do not report, but since they are Italy, Japan, Spain and Great Britain they can be expected to have low per capita costs of insurance and administration. The weighted average of the reporting comparison nations, including Germany, is $91.80 per capita. Without Germany it is $53.24. If the other comparison nations have this same average, then all of the comparison nations combined would average $69.49. This would be 32% of the American total. For comparison I believe we should not include Germany since their system is making similar mistakes in utilizing multiple insurance payments. The other comparison nations are spending about 24% of what Americans are spending for insurance underwriting and administration. The excess paid by Americans is estimated at 76% of the total recorded in 1998 or $43.9 billion. This is $428 per household or $165 per capita.

Excess Administration Costs of Providers

The insurance and administrative costs tracked by the OECD are the direct costs. The multiple private insurance companies, HMOs and government insurance programs in America dump as much of their administration as they can on the doctors' offices, hospitals and other providers. These are costs paid as part of hospital billings or doctors' fees. Some physicians and groups believe that half of their administrative costs are excessive. Our interviewers found similar complaints in Germany.

In Germany, the doctors complained about burdensome bureaucracy. The figures confirm that there is waste. Obviously American doctors, and as you know I am no exception, also complain of bureaucracy, which consumes a lot of time and money in the United States. One published estimate is that healthcare administration, overhead, paperwork and bureaucracy consume twenty-four cents of every U.S. healthcare dollar.[22]

The comparison to determine the excess expense in the U.S. should be against a single-payer program. Canada has a simplified billing and collecting mechanism demonstrating how single-payer nations lower administrative costs. Canadian doctors are reported to experience administrative costs of 10% of their billings, all of which they collect. In U.S. doctors' offices the sum of administrative costs generally is estimated at half of the difference between revenue and the doctor's income. The other half is for nursing, equipment, occupancy, utilities and insurance. Total doctors' revenue in 1998 was $229 billion. The expenses were estimated to be $122.5 billion. Half of this spent on administration would be $61.2 billion. But, Canadian experience would expect administration to be $22.9 billion. This would indicate an excess cost in the U.S. of $38.3 billion. Allowing Americans an extra 20% of this amount, the excess for American doctors' offices would be $31 billion, or $302 per household.

The excess administration from multiple insurance payers also affects the hospitals. The only ready means of measuring the possible excess is to compare the activity. In 1998 there were 829 million visits to physicians' offices in the United States and 75 million outpatient visits to hospitals. There were 31.8 million discharges of inpatients from hospitals.[23] The hospitals handled about 13% as many individuals as the doctors, but they have much more complex patients to treat. Another indication is employment. There were 1,803,000 employees in doctors' offices and clinics and 3,926,000 employees in hospitals. With these statistics in mind it is a reasonable assumption that the costs of excess administration in hospitals is around one half of that in doctors' offices. This is $15.5 billion or about $152 per household. The combined total of excess administrative costs in 1998 on U.S. providers is therefore estimated at $46.5 billion. This is $456 per household.

The total of excess costs of insurance, HMOs and the administrative burden they place on doctors and hospitals is estimated to have been $89.5 billion in 1998. This is $877 per household or $331 per person and more than 1% of American GDP. The healthcare lobby doesn't talk about this horrendous waste. Most Americans could find a better way to spend $331.

Medical equipment

The latest data comparing nations in terms of particular medical equipment units per million of population is from 1997:[24]

Selected Medical Equipment per Million of Population (OECD 2000)

	CAT scanners	MRIs	Radiation therapy units	Lithotriptors	Dialysis stations
Australia	–	–	4.9	7.5	–
Canada	8.2	1.8	7.0	0.5	59.6
France	9.7	2.5	7.7	0.8	168.5
Germany	17.1	6.2	4.6	1.7	–
Italy	14.8	4.1	2.4	–	158.1
Japan	69.7	18.0	4.0	–	–
Netherlands	9.0	3.9	–	0.8	–
Spain	9.3	4.1	2.4	1.8	–
United Kingdom	6.1	4.3	–	–	24.3
Switzerland	18.3	12.4	11.1	3.5	8.2
USA	13.7	7.6	4.3	2.3	–

Another study from this same year showed just CAT scanners and MRIs and included data for Japan and Great Britain. Japan was a little ahead of the U.S., and Great Britain was lower than the European countries shown here.[25]

Neither the referenced study or the OECD data includes the newest equipment, such as PET scans, fiber optic based diagnostic and surgical instruments, and other advanced surgical or therapeutic equipment. It would be difficult to assume equality between the U.S. and Europe; it is likely that the U.S. is better equipped. It is a much larger area with isolated communities. But, extra equipment is not always a benefit. If doctors' groups invest in equipment such as x-ray machines, they tend to use them. That gives them extra income, sometimes from unnecessary treatment or diagnostic are probably best done outside doctors' offices to mitigate temptation for over utilization.

While it is assumed that the U.S. has more diagnostic and therapeutic equipment, the OECD provides statistics of the number of hospital beds per thousand of population. The United States and Canada have about the same: 4 and 4.2. In Germany and France, however, the number is 9.4 and 8.5.[26] Hospitalization is far more expensive in the United States than in the comparison countries. According to the OECD statisticians, hospital cost per day in the United States is $1,128, in Canada it is $489, in France $284, in Germany $228.[27]

Equipment expense includes depreciation and maintenance, and replacement items or consumables. Hospital administrators in the U.S. generally allow ten to twelve percent of their budgets to pay for the various items of equipment and maintenance. If we assume that the U.S. has 50% more equipment than the comparison nations, then four percent of the total billings by hospitals ($382.8 billion) or $15.2 billion would be the hospital equipment share of the differential of excess cost. Physicians and their groups are estimated to have an equipment maintenance and consumables expense of 5% of the billings. If American doctors have twice the equipment of their OECD counterparts this would add $5.7 billion of excess. The total excess costs for diagnostic, therapeutic and surgical equipment would be $20.9 billion, or $205 per household.

The Lawyers

The advertising of plaintiff lawyers on billboards, in phone books, in newspapers and on television reminds doctors several times a day of the threat of lawsuits. In 1991, the average U.S. doctor was sued once every seven years, while the average Canadian doctor was sued once every fifty years.[28] With the real and perceived threat of plaintiff lawyers and litigation, doctors practice "defensive medicine" and order extra tests, consultations and medications to "cover their hides" and "make sure they don't miss anything." There is no clear data concerning this item on the American medical budget. AMA surveys indicate that the annual cost of malpractice insurance is $9 billion. The common assumption is that 10% of all medical tests and related diagnostic services are done because of the fear of what might happen in depositions or in a courtroom.

The Census of Business shows the1998 revenues of medical testing laboratories to be $15.2 billion. In 1998 U.S. hospitals performed 17,720,000 diagnostic or non-surgical procedures on inpatients. It is not clear what the hospitals' total charge was for all of these tests and procedures. What is clear is that the threat of possible law suits costs money. Along with the insurance company and HMO reviewers, there seems to be a lawyer in every examining room and operating room across America.

We have to assume that the cost of defensive medicine is substantial. Ten percent of the doctors' revenues in 1998 would be $22.9 billion. Adding the cost of the insurance would bring the total to $31.9 billion. This is $312 per household. There are no comparable costs in Europe, where the loser in a lawsuit pays the legal expenses of the winner.

Medical Research

The United States does spend the most money in the world on research and development (R&D) in the field of medicine. The healthcare lobby frequently uses this fact in its arguments to prevent the enactment of a national health program. Total spending in the U.S. on R&D in 1998 is estimated at nearly $42 billion. The public funded portion was $19.9 billion.[29] Pharmaceutical industry R&D was estimated at over $22 billion.[30]

I believe this excess spending in the U.S. is worthwhile for the most part, especially if we are developing new technologies, therapies or medications that actually make a real difference in preventing diseases or in treating patients. The U.S. is also the wealthiest nation in the world. In terms of medical research spending, the true world leaders are the wealthy nations, for they have the financial means to invest in these important areas. The American excess of public funded research was 63% higher than in the reporting comparison nations on a per capita basis. This indicates an excess expense of $12.5 billion which Americans contributed to through tax payments.[31] There was also an excess of private research expenses, which Americans contributed to by buying drugs and medical services. This was 46% higher than the weighted average of the reporting comparison nations (except Italy and The Netherlands), which indicated an excess of $10.1 billion. The total of excess expenditure for research was $22.6 billion or $222 per household.

Dental Costs

Most Americans realize the cost of dental care in the U.S. is expensive, but overall dental costs are probably not an excess expense relative to the comparison nations. When comparing our overall costs to the other nations, the U.S. possibly "under spends" for dental services. The U.S. total dentistry expense in 1998 was approximately 4.7% of total healthcare costs compared to other nations weighted average of 7.1%. Some nations spent up to 10% on dental care overall.[32] There may be no excess expenditure on dentistry by Americans, but I'm not sure that is a sound health policy. Over 90 million Americans (most of them without dental insurance) fail to see a dentist in any single year.[33]

Anomalies in the Reported Data

I have, with the Olin Frederick staff, worked extensively with the data provided by the Healthcare Policy Unit of the OECD located in Paris. It has been evident that there may be differences in reporting practices between different nations. An attempt is underway to meld the data into an International Classification of Health Accounts (ICHA). So far only Germany has recalculated data to this standard. There are more details in the reference about individual reporting practices. It is generally evident, however, that the United States, Canada, France, and Germany are probably about equal in reporting. There are some noted omissions of small significance by Great Britain, The Netherlands and Australia. Japan maintains that they include everything. Italy and Spain give no details. Considering this, it is good judgment to assume a portion of the apparent excess expense in the U.S. may be due to reporting differences in the comparison nations. The amount we have selected is 20% of the average expenditure on healthcare of the comparison nations, which was 103.1 billion. This adds $20.6 billion.

In previous chapters I spoke of the fraud that unfortunately occurs in healthcare in the form of dishonest and potentially harmful practices, and is costly to any society. The Office of Inspector General estimated fraudulent and erroneous claims cost Medicare $13.5 billion in 1999.[34] I can find no evidence that the amount of fraud in American medicine is more or less than the comparison nations. America's numerous payers and fragmented system, however, may be to the advantage of those who unfortunately practice this type of medicine. One colleague jokingly commented, "It is easier to steal billions from thousands of different sources and payers than to steal billions from one national health program."

This is a summary of these excess "American" costs of healthcare for 1998:

High marketing expenses in the pharmaceutical industry	$10.9 billion
Higher prices for prescription medications	13.7
Higher incomes for American physicians	53.4
Excessive costs of insurance by multi-payers	43.9
Excess administrative costs for providers	46.5
Cost of American level of diagnostic and therapeutic equipment	20.9
Cost of malpractice insurance and defensive medicine	31.9
More research per capita	22.6
Adjustment for reporting differences	20.6
Total	$ 264.4

Assuming these calculations are reasonably correct, the total differential in 1998 that we can account for in total healthcare costs is approximately $264.4 billion. This is the predictable American excess cost of healthcare as itemized versus the comparison countries. But, the actual differential between the U.S. and the comparison OECD countries is $428 billion. There is a gap in the differential. This is approximately $163.6 billion; about $1,595 per household and $606 per capita. This is the amount not explained by obviously high physicians' incomes, insurance costs and bureaucracy, hospital equipment costs, defensive medicine, more R&D or excess pharmaceutical industry marketing costs and higher drug prices.

This gap of over $160 billion in excess costs related to the comparison nations outside the predictors is the huge cost of caring for numerous sick Americans whose illnesses would have been prevented in the comparison nations under their universal healthcare systems. Patients in the United States who lack access to or experience delays in receiving appropriate primary and preventive care, end up being sicker in the long run and costing the system more. The lack of a universal national health policy in the United States allows people to get sick from lack of access to basic preventive and primary levels of care. In America, decent healthcare is not provided to all people as is called for in the United Nations declaration of 1948. The United States has yet to grant this basic human right to its people.

The financial cost of caring for the sick is enormous! *Consumer Reports* in September 2000 showed the costs of caring for the sickest 10% of Americans was $22,578 per person or $614 billion. According to the study, the healthiest 10% cost "nearly nothing."[35] Another study found 10% of the population using 72% of the healthcare cost.[36] It has been reported that 4% of Medicare patients use 46% of Medicare costs, or over $63,000 per patient per year.[37] Studies show the sickest patients are also more likely to be poor, elderly, less educated, uninsured and of an ethnic minority. I hope, by now, that is not a surprise to anyone.

It is clear that the American system exacerbates its own high cost. It has more sick, lower income people than the comparison countries by a large margin. In the last ten years, this may have cost Americans around a trillion dollars in excess health spending. In human terms it is unconscionable. It is also an unconscionable burden on the lower and middle classes of the nation in economic terms.

THE SICK PEOPLE WHO SHOULD NOT BE SICK

The second way to prove that America has higher healthcare costs and a "gap" between it and the other comparison nations is examining the prevalence and incidence of serious illnesses between the United States and other nations. Numerous studies support the premise that Americans face more severe illnesses compared to people of other wealthy countries that provide universal healthcare and insurance.

Preventive Care

In the early 1990s less than 5% of all healthcare expenditures were invested in the prevention of illness and disease in the U.S.[38] This is a poor market-driven strategy for this nation. For instance, only 74% of all American children have completed their recommended immunizations by the age of three.[39] I know we will never reach 100% immunizations in this nation, for there are some people who object to their use for religious, philosophical or personal reasons. However, cost and lack of insurance are the greatest barriers to childhood immunizations in the U.S. Immunizations have made a huge difference in the world's health. Small pox has been eliminated and common childhood killers such as measles are unheard of in the wealthy countries of the world. Unfortunately measles is still a common killer in third world countries. According to the Center for Disease Control (CDC), the nations of Canada, Finland, Netherlands, Sweden, U.K., and Japan provide greater measles immunization coverage rates compared to the U.S. rate of 91%.[40]

Preventive care is also important in adult medicine. This includes regular check-ups and screening tests. It also includes intervention in addictions and mental disorders. And perhaps most important of all, it means prompt action at the onset of symptoms. George, the carpenter, couldn't do anything about his early symptoms. Roy, the farmer, went to alternative medicine when he couldn't afford allopathic treatment. Both patients became expensive tragedies, as have millions of others. According to this 1998 survey of uninsured adults, between ages eighteen and sixty-four, over 2 million Americans in fair or poor health are estimated to not have seen any doctor in the previous year due to cost. Over 16 million adult patients failed to see any doctor for one year because of high costs and/or inadequate insurance according to this same study.[41] Obviously these people are not receiving many proven and effective preventive health measures.

Prenatal Care

In 1998 there were 3.940,000 live births in the U.S. Nearly 18% of pregnant women in the U.S. failed to obtain early prenatal care in their first trimester, and 3.9% of pregnant women received only late prenatal care or none at all.[42] Many mothers and newborns will suffer unnecessary consequences if such health services are delayed. In the other OECD nations that have universal healthcare, a woman giving birth without full prenatal care is extremely rare. See Figure Fifteen. Early prenatal care is clearly related to better patient and

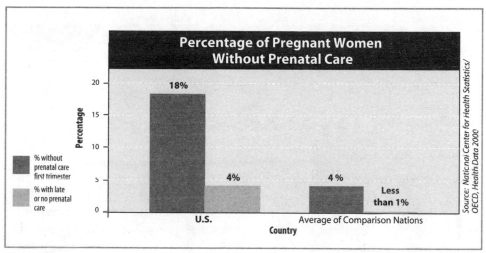

Figure Fifteen

infant outcomes. The estimated rate of preterm babies in the comparison nations has been between 5 and 10%. In 1999, the preterm delivery rate nationally in the U.S. was 11%. The medical costs of one premature baby alone can range from $20,000 to over $1 million.

A study by the Institute of Medicine demonstrated that every one dollar spent on prenatal care and education lowered future costs by three dollars.[42] Another study showed for every dollar cut in prenatal care cost, the postnatal long-term costs would increase by $4.63.[43] These facts are real. Mothers receiving early prenatal care have fewer complications related to the baby's delivery and also deliver fewer premature babies. The numbers of 18% and 3.9% may seem small to a healthcare lobbyist opposing universal health insurance, but the costs are enormous to the society. In the United States nearly 700,000 babies are born without first trimester care, and about 150,000 are born without any significant prenatal care. About 25% more American babies are born with low birth weight than in the comparison nations. This amounts to 58,000 babies. The average hospital stay for a baby with a perinatal condition is 10 days.[44] This suggests an average cost of at least $20,000. Low birth weight is not the only condition that might have to be treated because of inadequate prenatal attention.

The excess cost of low birth weight babies alone is $1.1 billion. The referenced study showing a loss of $4.63 per dollar of healthcare withheld from pregnant women suggests, for the 3.9% of mothers who forego prenatal care, the eventual cost is $2.5 billion. This is an average of $16,600 per baby.

There is also another measure. The infant mortality rate in the U.S. was 7.2 per 1,000 live births in 1997. See Figure Two on the next page. That was 19% more than the weighted average of the comparison nations using the

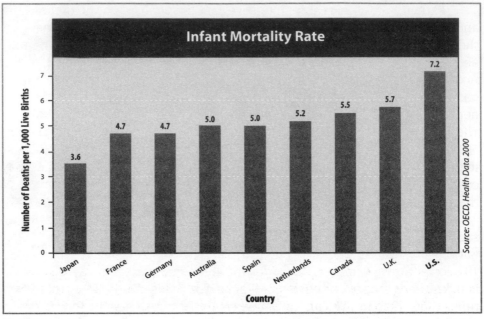

Figure Two

latest year reported.[45] For mothers, the rate of death was 8.4 per 100,000 births or 72% more than the comparison nations. The difference between the U.S. and the comparison nations was 191 more mothers and 4,561 more babies. Who would like to put a price on these human lives? Universal healthcare providing prenatal care for all women in the U.S. would cost less than the excess perinatal treatments and the human losses.

Acute Respiratory Failure

Americans, young and old, face more episodes of acute respiratory failure (ARF) much more frequently than Europeans, according to two European studies.[46, 47] Many suffer the consequences of untreated asthma, high blood pressure, pneumonia, and heart failure in the U.S. and present to emergency rooms gasping for air. Sam, the farmer whose story is in Chapter One, was an example. These conditions are oftentimes treatable and preventable. A 1994 U.S. nationwide inpatient sample estimated ARF at 137.1 per 100,000 residents aged five years and older.[48] A 1995 German study estimated ARF of 110.8 per 100,000 residents aged fourteen years and older.[49] Another European survey of ARF yielded a much lower estimate of 77.6 per 100,000 population aged fifteen years and older.[50] Even adjusting for the slight age differences, Americans suffer more respiratory failure compared to the European countries with universal coverage.

Patients with ARF require intensive care hospitalization with ventilators and other lifesaving measures. The European studies show that many of these expensive hospitalizations probably could be prevented with afford-able and accessible healthcare and prescription coverage as an outpatient. According to a 1995 U.S. national health survey, disabling asthma in children has more than doubled since 1969.[51] Asthma tends to strike the most vul-nerable of our children and society; the poor, less educated and smokers. The U.S. may have at least 20% more cases of ARF per 100,000 people and 50,000 excess intensive care hospital admissions. If the average hospital cost in the U.S. for ARF is $40,000, which the available data suggests, then we pay over $2 billion dollars in excessive costs related to our under-treatment of these chronic and treatable conditions.[52]

Americans also have more potential years of life lost before age seventy secondary to chronic obstructive pulmonary disease (COPD). Among the ten nations, the death rate is greatest in the U.S. compared to approximately 10% lower rates in the U.K., Canada, and Australia. The American death rate is three times that of Germany and France, ten times that of Italy and twenty times that of Japan. We cannot blame cigarette smoking since the compari-son nations have 34% more daily smokers on average.[53] See Figure Sixteen.

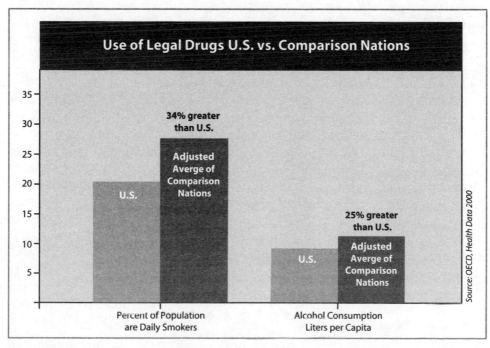

Figure Sixteen

In 1993 the direct medical cost of COPD was estimated at $14.7 billion.[54] If the comparison nations have a 20% lower rate of COPD, the U.S. may be facing excess costs of over $2.9 billion. The 1998 consumer price index is approximately 20% higher than 1993 prices. Combined with ARF this nation may have $5.9 billion in excess direct respiratory related costs relative to the comparison nations.

Uncovered and untreated diseases such as asthma, chronic bronchitis, hypertension, and heart failure are costly in human terms and costly in later medical expenses. Sadly, many Americans die much younger from respiratory illness, a fate of those people in nations without decent health insurance and access to timely care.

Mental Illness

Americans may also suffer from more mental disorders compared to other similar countries such as The Netherlands, Germany, or Canada. The WHO (World Health Organization) International Consortium in Psychiatric Epidemiology examined data from these countries and found people experienced at least one mental disorder in their lifetime in 48% of those studied in the U.S., compared to 40% in The Netherlands, 38% in Germany, and 37% in Canada.[55] The researchers found mental disorders becoming more frequent, often beginning in early teenage years and afflicting many people for a lifetime. They also found nearly one-half of those with mental disorders fail to seek psychiatric help, and many others are not even treated, even though effective therapies exist. Part of primary care is to spot the precursors of mental illness. It is very important to recognize that mental illness is a disease like arthritis or diabetes and can be managed with proper treatment. In 1990 the cost of depression in the U.S. was estimated at $43 billion per year with 30% related to direct medical costs.[57] The U.S. has a 20% higher incidence of depression relative to the comparison nations, and Americans may face excess costs of over $8 billion (1990 dollars) partly because of the failure to provide universal mental health services and parity. In 1998, the price index in the U.S. increased by 27% over 1990. This suggests the excess cost of mental illness in 1998 was $10 billion.

Emergency Rooms for the Uninsured

Another hidden additional cost on the American healthcare system is high emergency room expenses, partially related to lack of adequate access for uninsured Americans. Studies show emergency room services account for "only 2%" of the nation's healthcare expenditures.[58] This, however, amounts to $23 billion annually. Uninsured people frequently use the emergency rooms as their source of medical care. For instance, in the Maryland Health

Initiative, uninsured citizens represented 14% of the state's population, but accounted for 23% of the emergency room visits from 1997 to 1999.[59] Outpatient physician office visits easily cost less than half that of an ER visit. If we assume that the uninsured would have ER utilization rates similar to the insured citizens under a universal health insurance program, potentially 9% of all ER visits presently are excess expense. This may cost the system nearly $2.1 billion in excess costs. But, even if the proponents of the market-driven system think the ER is a solution for uninsured people they are terribly wrong. The ER does not provide preventive or primary care and essentially, no continuity of care. And, when uninsured people become ER patients they are usually sick. A primary goal of medicine is to keep people from getting sick.

Diabetes

Diabetes is one of the most expensive, frequent, and serious chronic diseases. Both the direct and indirect U.S. costs of diabetes in 1998 were estimated at $92 billion. One out of every five Americans will suffer this disease before the age of seventy. Those in the lowest socioeconomic class face death rates twice as high compared with the highest socioeconomic class.[59] Nearly one-half of the increased risk of death in the lowest social group was accounted for by other risk factors such as high blood pressure and smoking. Access to adequate healthcare and insurance may have significantly influenced these rates, since high blood pressure and nicotine addiction are treatable.

Multiple medical studies have shown that the treatment of diabetes leads to improved quality of life and less chronic complications for the patient. One study showed that for every $1 spent on diabetes education there was a $2-$3 cost savings from reduced diabetic hospitalizations.[60] Another recent medical study showed that improved diabetic control leads to lower healthcare costs and saves money.[61] However, those patients in the study had decent health insurance with affordable medications. In my community, one out of five working-age adults has no insurance. Well over one-third of the 39 million Medicare beneficiaries have no insurance with which to pay for prescription drugs outside the hospital.[62] A Congressional Budget Office study estimated the average Medicare beneficiary prescription costs were $1,525 for each patient in 2000.[63] This book is replete with patients who have suffered the consequences of untreated and under-treated diabetes over their lifetime. It costs infinitely more to let diabetics go under-treated early on and then try to correct the unfortunate consequences later. Believe me when I say that George, the diabetic carpenter, and others, truly had rotten toes and feet from their lack of health coverage.

The death rate and potential years of life lost before age seventy in the U.S. was higher than any of the comparison nations in 1998. The statistics showed the U.S. death rate was three times that of France, Japan and Great Britain, twice that of Spain, 20% higher than Canada and the Netherlands, 15% higher than Germany, and 10% higher than Italy. Death rates from diabetes in the weighted average of the comparison nations were 43% lower than the U.S. or 11.8 versus 20.9 per 100,000 people respectively.[65] The U.S. also has drastically higher potential life years lost before age seventy from this disease: five times more than France, three times more than Japan, Great Britain and Spain, two and a half times more than Australia and double Germany, Italy and The Netherlands. Diabetic Americans are not guaranteed health insurance until they receive Medicare at age sixty-five and this helps to produce these undesirable, sad outcomes. Hardworking Americans die younger from diabetes.[66]

The U.S. has more young patients who develop severe symptoms earlier and who will require extended treatment. The comparison nations have less of the severe symptoms, or fewer patients who are sick with the disease and die from it. The excess cost paid by Americans cannot be less than double that of the comparison nations, which was $45.5 billion, but it is most likely more. Averaging the excesses calculates to an excess expense of $55.2 billion in 1998, more than one half of one percent of GDP. There are numerous diabetics trying to cope with their disease without adequate resources. Over 1.5 million known diabetics are uninsured for over one year, and I estimate that over three million Medicare diabetics lack decent prescription coverage.[67]

A recent survey estimated that about five million Americans are unaware that they have diabetes. Would anyone care to speculate as to why? It is hard to make the diagnosis when you lack health insurance and fail to see a doctor. Americans also have more diabetes because of obesity. The comparison nations have 44% less diabetes cases than the U.S. We are becoming more and more sedentary as a society and are now facing some of the unhealthy consequences. Obese patients' access to medical care can help them realize the importance of regular exercise and diet.

It will be impossible to rein in health costs in this nation if common and deadly diseases such as diabetes and obesity are allowed to go untreated.

Kidney Failure

More diabetic Americans per million of population are on dialysis. In 1994 the yearly incidence of end stage renal disease (ESRD) with diabetes was significantly greater in the U.S. (107 cases) per million people, nearly two-to-eight times greater when compared to Japan (66.0), Australia (14.0), Norway (15.4), Germany (52.0) or Italy (13.0).[68] See Figure Seventeen. The vast majority of ESRD patients are treated with very expensive treatments including dialysis

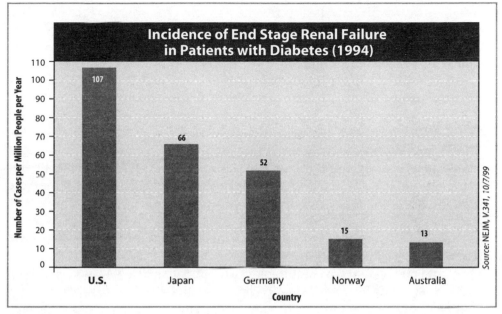

Figure Seventeen

and renal transplants. ESRD cost $12 billion in the U.S. in 1998, with an average hemodialysis patient costing $48,207 per year.[69] African-American patients are five times more likely than whites to need dialysis. Because minority populations are more likely to be uninsured than white Americans, the minorities also suffer more from the consequences of untreated diabetes and high blood pressure. African-Americans have a greater predisposition to hypertension. Of all ESRD patients, 64% are related to two chronic conditions, diabetes and high blood pressure.[70] Over time, these untreated chronic conditions lead to progressive loss of kidney function and eventually ESRD, which is costly to all Americans. Medicare covers 100% of the people on dialysis. The comparison nations have 62% fewer deaths from ESRD and 23% fewer people on dialysis compared to the U.S.[71] By providing universal coverage, the comparison nations had one-half the incidence of ESRD in 1994, making an excess cost of $6 billion.

Peripheral Vascular Disease

With untreated diabetes and high blood pressure, patients can also develop peripheral vascular disease, heart disease and strokes, all major causes of chronic disabilities and/or death. Peripheral vascular disease frequently leads to amputations. A recent study published in 2000, compared the incidence of major amputations in a U.S. community to communities in other countries with universal health insurance, including four in England, and one each in Japan, Italy, Taiwan, and Spain. The community in the U.S. had yearly amputation rates per 100,000 population of nineteen for men and twelve for women. This compares to the other countries averages of fifteen for men or six for women in England, seven for men or five for women in Italy, three for men or one for women in Japan, eight for men or six for women in Taiwan, and three for men or one for women in Spain.[72] If we assume the U.S. has a higher incidence of major amputations at four for men and six for women per 100,000 in relation to the comparison nations, we may suffer 14,000 excess major amputations secondary to our lack of a universal care system. This probably costs all Americans another $1 billion yearly, not to mention the devastating loss of limbs and the suffering and societal cost of possible permanent disability.

Some may argue that the U.S. doesn't have more amputations compared to other nations, but try telling that to chronically uninsured, Lillian, a patient I met recently in the emergency room. She had a history of diabetes and earlier in her life had insurance and a doctor. But, she lost her job and health insurance five years ago when a local manufacturing plant closed. Lillian then lived with and cared for her mother who was ill with cancer and eventually succumbed to the illness. Over the next few years Lillian then cared for her sister who was mentally retarded from a birth defect. These two sisters over the ensuing years lived on a total income of $722 per month combined. However, diabetic Lillian remained uninsured and was even denied Medicaid benefits. Our irrational healthcare system denied her health insurance because she had IRA funds from her previous employment. The long standing diabetic failed to see any doctor or dentist for many years because of her lack of insurance and the potential high costs should she seek care.

In my opinion, what happened to Lillian cost her and society far more than simply covering her with universal insurance years earlier. Lillian "stubbed" her toe and waited two days before coming to the ER. The pain and swelling of her foot became unbearable. I was called to see her for a medical consultation concerning her various problems. When I walked into the examination room, the smell of the swollen and ulcerated foot was overwhelming. There was obvious gangrene of the foot, and she suffered from severe dehydration and uncontrolled diabetes. Lillian had acid in the blood stream, another life-threatening problem from lack of insulin. She also had lost over twenty pounds from dehydration and untreated diabetes and looked at least twenty years older than her stated age. The emergency room staff and I soon stabilized her and she was taken quickly to the operating room where a surgeon performed a below-the-knee amputation. As her treating doctors, we knew there was no hope of saving her leg. This uninsured diabetic's first health system encounter in nearly five years was an emergency amputation. That is what happened to Americans living prior to the discovery of insulin in the 1920s. Why is this still happening in the United States today?

Lillian's critical illness was preventable with any reasonable access to healthcare. I know this illness has already cost over $40,000, for she has shown me her bills. And potentially even greater costs will follow as her kidney function and eyesight have already shown decline. The chances of Lillian needing dialysis are well over 50% in the next five years, assuming she survives.

Where are the presumed cost savings in America by denying this patient comprehensive health insurance years ago? Is it not cost that is the major barrier to our nation implementing a universal system? Does anyone really count the additional costs of untreated illness, preventable disabilities and early deaths this society suffers for their lack of a national health policy? For now society and Lillian must cope with her new disability and also a disabled sister. What will happen to Lillian's impaired sister if she loses her caregiver? Will she find herself living in a government-supported group home?

Let me reflect reality on the healthcare lobby line and others who "blame the patient." Lillian did not smoke, drink alcohol or use drugs. She is a real person and was a productive member of her family and society. She loved and cared for her mother and sister. Uninsured Americans lose more than just their legs.

Sometimes I think the U.S. system supports "Social Darwinism": that is let the poor, less educated, or chronically ill people suffer and die prematurely. The reality is that every job is important. Good janitors mean there are clean rest rooms. Good garbage collectors mean there are clean neighborhoods. Good farm hands means productive farms and cheap food. All through the books of the great religions, the well-to-do are exhorted to look after the poor people of their society. What has happened to the traditional social consciousness of Americans?

Dental Care

As previously stated 90 million Americans fail to see a dentist each year, and most of these people have no dental insurance. Why are the dentists in America not screaming in protest with so many people failing to obtain such basic dental health needs?

American studies have shown dental loss is significantly correlated with age, lower income, less education, lack of insurance, and smoking. And edentulism, the loss of all natural permanent teeth, causes a significant lowering of a person's quality of life, self-image, and daily functioning. Those without dental insurance had a 50% higher rate of edentulism.[72] Fluoridation of drinking water can significantly reduce dental cavities and future dental loss, available to over 50% of the U.S. population in 1999. Fluoridation of drinking water safely and inexpensively prevents tooth decay for children and adults regardless of socioeconomic status or access to care. Over the previous forty-five years fluoridation helped reduce tooth decay 40 to 70% in children and tooth loss 40 to 60% in adults, saving billions yearly in potential future dental related costs.[73] Yet, over 100 million Americans still drink water without these benefits.

I had difficulty finding actual head-to-head international studies comparing the incidence of dental loss between the U.S. and other countries. In the U.S. unpublished CDC 1999 data showed that 9.1% of persons aged forty-five to fifty-four years were edentulous. In a forty-six-state survey in the U.S. of 28,979 persons aged sixty-five years and older, edentulism ranged from 13.9% in Hawaii to 47.9% in West Virginia. Only five states had rates less than 20% (Arizona, California, Hawaii, Oregon, and Wisconsin).[74] One Swedish study examined adults with teeth over an eighteen-year period and found a tooth loss rate of 0.2 to 2.6 for age groups between twenty and sixty, and well less than 2% edentulous for older Swedes.[75] I understand dental health insurance and access to dental services are significantly better in Sweden and Hawaii as compared to the rest of America. The costs of unfluoridated water and lack of universal dental insurance are enormous in the U.S. But who is counting all the missing teeth?

One day a patient of mine, a dentist, told me how busy his practice was now. He just joined a state dental insurance program, Child Health Insurance Program (CHIP), for children. The vast majority of children in our county and this country have no dental health insurance. He told me, "Many children are now coming in with rotten teeth; it's awful." He seemed pleased that he could finally help these unfortunate children. But then he told me how difficult it is for Medicaid patients to obtain a dental appointment in our community. Our county, among the largest in land acreage in New York State, has only three dentists participating with CHIP or Medicaid. This makes dental access to the poor and children in our county much more difficult with another long waiting line.

Poor dental healthcare outcomes may also affect other diseases including cardiac and cerebral vascular diseases. Recent studies show patients with periodontal disease and edentulism having 66% and 23% higher risks of strokes respectively.[77] Again, who is counting the greater numbers of strokes?

Stroke

In 1991 a report of the Task Force on Research in Epidemiology and Prevention of Cardiovascular Diseases found cardiovascular death rates had declined significantly over time in the U.S. But these figures show that Americans still suffered from these serious diseases much more commonly than many of the countries already mentioned. American men died from cardiovascular diseases at nearly 500 per 100,000 that year. Australia, The Netherlands, Canada, Italy, Spain, Japan and France each had lower cardiovascular death rates for men and women compared to the U.S. population. Japanese and French males had less than 250 per 100,000 deaths from stroke.[78]

A study published in 1998 estimated Americans suffered more than 700,000 strokes.[79] Estimates on the long-term costs of strokes average from $46,000 (minor) to $124,000 (major).[80] Assuming the average stroke cost is $85,000 and one-quarter of strokes are preventable with universal healthcare, the U.S. spends nearly $15 billion in excess stroke costs for lack of a decent health system.[81]

Heart Failure

Nearly five million Americans (1.8% of the total) suffer from congestive heart failure (CHF), a serious disabling and life-threatening disease. For those over sixty-five years of age, the prevalence increases to 6-10% and is the leading cause of hospitalization in this age group. Direct medical costs related to CHF are estimated at $20-40 billion per year. The four most common causes of CHF are coronary artery disease (60%), cigarette smoking (17%), high blood pressure (10%) and lack of physical activity (9%).[82] Major risk factors for coronary artery disease are diabetes and high cholesterol, which are preventable and treatable.

I could not find large international studies showing the prevalence of CHF in the comparison nations. However, a Swedish study estimated their population suffered CHF at 2.8% for those aged 65–74 and 6.1% for those aged 75–79.[83] I estimate their entire population may have a prevalence of 1.0%, which is significantly less than the U.S. According to 1991 data, American men had 25% and women had 46% higher cardiovascular death rates for those in the 35–74 age groups in relation to the average of the comparison nations.[84] The U.S. probably has at least a 25% higher prevalence of heart failure when compared to these other nations on average and may be facing excessive costs amounting to $5–10 billion per year. We face these serious illnesses largely because we leave so many diabetic, hypertensive and high-cholesterol patients without affordable medications and decent health insurance coverage that assures adequate physician monitoring.

The OECD Health Policy Unit lumps statistics of heart disease and stroke into a category of "diseases of the circulatory system" with two other categories of "acute myocardial infarction" and "ischemic heart disease." In the generalized category in 1997 the United States was 30% higher than the weighted average of the comparison nations in death rate per 100,000 and 60 percent higher in potential years of life lost before age 70. The statistics for the myocardial infarctions showed the U.S. in 1997 as 23% higher in death rate and 32% higher in potential life years lost before age 70 versus the weighted average of the comparison nations. The American death rate by ischemic heart disease was 53% higher than the weighted average of the comparison nations and 67% higher in potential years of life lost before age seventy.[85] In circulatory or heart diseases, Americans die younger than in other diseases we have measured.

The total direct costs of all cardiovascular diseases in the U.S. were estimated at $127 billion in 1995, or 17% of total healthcare costs. Hospitalizations accounted for 50% of the costs, and nursing homes accounted for 20%.[86] In 1998 at 17% of total healthcare costs, cardiovascular disease would have been $195 billion. Judging by the OECD data there are at least 50% more seriously ill patients in the U.S. than in Europe and Japan, pro-rated by population. This means that at least 33% of the cost of these diseases should have been avoided and is excess. This is estimated at $64.3 billion with the 1995 results transposed into 1998, correcting for healthcare inflation.

No wonder this nation needs more specialists. We leave millions of people with diabetes, high blood pressure, and high cholesterol untreated. Thankfully, the death rates from major cardiovascular diseases have been falling in the U.S., as well as in the comparison nations. In the U.S., rates from these diseases have steadily fallen since the 1960s, corresponding to the enactment of Medicare and Medicaid by President Lyndon Johnson.[87] (See Figure Eighteen) However, the U.S. decline in death rates have leveled off some in the 1990s and are falling at a slower rate than the comparison nations.[88] This nation will continue to have difficulty further reducing mortality rates from cardiovascular diseases as long as we leave up to 40% of Medicare patients without decent prescription coverage and 43 million Americans without health insurance. Affordable insurance and medications for all Americans will save countless patients from premature death, disability, unnecessary hospitalizations and nursing home placements along with the high costs.

HIV/AIDS

HIV/AIDS is a devastating disease to the infected patients, their families and society. Worldwide an estimated 36.1 million people are infected with HIV and over 22 million people have died from AIDS.[89] The incidence of AIDS in the U.S. was 17.1 per 100,000 people in 1998.[90] However this rate can vary

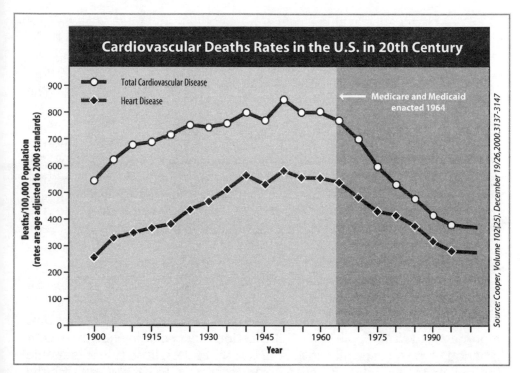

Figure Eighteen

among the states from a low of 0.6 in North Dakota to 39.4 in New York. The District of Columbia had 189.4 cases per 100,000 people in a one-year period ending mid-2000.[91]

I know the U.S. health system fails to offer parity or even minimally decent treatment to all people suffering from drug abuse and addictions. Illegal intravenous drug use has been estimated to cause approximately 30% of the AIDS cases. I have seen these patients in my community and elsewhere go untreated for years. I believe we all pay a heavy price for this shallow-minded health policy. The U.S. has eight times the incidence of AIDS of the weighted average of the comparison nations.[92] Health costs alone for treating this illness as a result of drug abuse has been further estimated at $4.4 billion in 1999 direct costs.[93] Untreated drug abuse with resulting AIDS is estimated to cost this nation over $3.8 billion in excess direct medical costs in relation to the comparison nations.

How do the wealthy nations compare in their efforts to stop this deadly "plague" of the 20th and 21st centuries? According to this report, Japan committed $3 billion a year to the "Global Fund" to fight worldwide HIV/AIDS. Somehow the U.S. can only muster $200 million for this same purpose.[94] Some congressional leaders later promised another $1.3 billion.[95] But will this wise investment ever pass the Congress and be signed by the President?

Compared to Japan, America has nearly twice the population, has far more drug abuse, and twenty times the number of HIV/AIDS patients. What is the U.S. reluctance to support the struggle against this deadly disease in the world?

HIV/AIDS is treatable, and deaths have fallen in the U.S. from 50,610 in 1995 to 16,273 in 1999.[96] "Triple drug" therapy has made a great difference in extending the life of AIDS patients, but it costs about $10,000 per patient per year in the U.S. Somehow "triple therapy" prices are possible in some foreign countries at $350 per patient per year.[97] The American pharmaceutical industry has the potential to lower prices for the American people and also the world. America cannot claim to be the greatest nation in the world when we turn our backs on this disease in our own homeland and in Africa. Ironically, the highest incidence of HIV/AIDS occurs in the nation's capital city where the people with the power to implement a national health program work and govern.

Disabilities

Untreated chronic diseases of every kind can lead to disabling health conditions at enormous costs. The cost of disabilities from diabetes alone is estimated at $37.1 billion in 1997 for the U.S.[98] An OECD Health Data 2000 report showed that people of all OECD nations are becoming healthier. Over a period of thirty years, all OECD countries have decreased their premature mortality rates by one-half and this rate continues to drop. In the United States, on the other hand, this premature death rate is still 20% higher for men and 11% higher for women compared to the average OECD nation. Compared to these other countries, the U.S. has the highest rate of premature death and the most potential years of life lost before age 70 per 100,000 people (6,496), almost twice the number of Japan (3,421).[99] Refer to Figure One on page 115.

Not only do Americans die prematurely, but they also face more disability and at a younger age. Untreated common medical conditions lead to chronic disability: blindness, amputations, paralysis, breathing problems, mental illness or health conditions related to premature births. This is measured by Disability Adjusted Life Years (DALY). These are the sums of life years lost due to premature mortality and years lived with disability adjusted for severity.[100] See Figures Nineteen and Twenty.

The U.S. is far behind many of the OECD nations in DALY statistics. According to the 2000 *World Health Report*, the U.S. ranked 24th in the world in DALY estimates. Worldwide, the comparison nations' rankings are as follows: Japan—first, France—third, Spain—fifth, Italy—sixth, Canada—12th, The Netherlands—13th, Britain—14th and Germany—22nd.

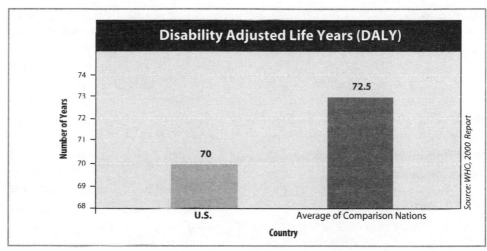

Figure Nineteen

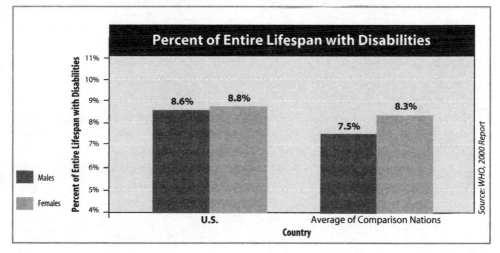

Figure Twenty

The Other Diseases

Two major diseases are missing from the list. The data for all types of cancer in the comparison nations shows the U.S. had a 2.8% higher death rate and was 1.8% higher in years lost versus the comparison nations. Cancer is one of the few diseases for which the OECD keeps incidence statistics, but the U.S. does not report. The comparison nations all have higher smoking rates. In the U.S. only 20.7% of the population were daily smokers in 1997, while Italy reported 25.7%, Spain 33.1% and The Netherlands 34.6%. Germany reported 26% and Australia 25.1% for 1995.; Canada reported 23.8% and

Great Britain 27% for 1998. France and Japan did not report. For cancer, the U.S. likely incurs some extra expense. There were 1,220,000 new cases in 2000.

The other missing major disease is arthritis. The OECD has little data on arthritis as it is not implicated in deaths as much as the others we have examined. The reported death rates from arthritis show the United States rate is about the same as the average of the comparison nations, but Americans lose twice the number of potential years of life lost before 70. Americans die younger from untreated arthritis.[101] This indicates some potential large excess expense, but to certify this conclusion would require further data.

The incidence of chronic diseases from the U.S. National Center for Health Statistics for 1996 are:

Arthritis	38,638,000
Hypertension	28,314,000
Heart Conditions	20,653,000
Asthma	14,596,000
Chronic bronchitis	14,150,000
Diabetes	7,627,000

The data below is for cancer, respiratory, digestive and endocrine diseases.

Diseases	Comparison Nations Weighted Average		United States		U.S. vs. Comparison Average	
	Mort. rate	Years lost	Mort. Rate	Years lost	Mortality	Years lost
Cancer, all types	182	1136.5	187.2	1157.9	5.2 / 2.86%	21.4 / 1.88%
Digestive system	32.1	202.7	26.5	214	(5.6) / (17.45%)	11.3 / 5.57%
Endocrine/Metabolic	15.6	176.4	33.8	341	18.2 /116.67%	164.6 / 93.31%
Respiratory, all types	58.1	148.5	68.8	242.1	10.7 / 18.42%	93.6 / 63.03%

The United States had a lower death rate than the comparison nations from digestive diseases by 17.5%, but it was clear that Americans were dying younger, as the potential years of life lost before seventy by Americans was 11.3% higher. Americans died more often and younger than in the comparison nations from respiratory diseases. They had very high rates of endocrine diseases, but with a higher difference in the death rate than in years lost.

I do not have cost estimates for every serious disease and illness nor disability costs in the U.S. and the comparison nations. The evidence is strong, however, that there is more excess expenditure versus the comparison nations. How much we cannot tell, but will anyone bet that it was less than $11 billion in 1998? The summary of the excess cost paid by Americans due to the denial of primary and preventive care to all people living in this nation is:

Complications related to birth	$ 2.5 billion
Acute Respiratory Failure	5.9
Mental Illnesses	10.0
Emergency Room	2.1
Diabetes	55.2
End Stage Renal Disease	6.0
Cardiovascular diseases	64.3
HIV/AIDS and illegal drug use	3.4
Total	$149.4 billion

More statistics may be found in Figures Twenty-one through Twenty-three found on pages 166 and 167. Some may argue that these numbers are inaccurate and claim our system is far superior to the average comparison nations. However, I am not surprised by our poor performance, because I have seen too many Americans suffer from lack of a decent and just health system. America can lower these high and unnecessary costs of illnesses and reduce human suffering if Congress enacts a comprehensive national health program that covers all of the people all of the time.

A third clue to proving this gap of $160 billion in paying for excessive illness can be found in an analysis of the American population and the consumption of healthcare costs. See Figure Twenty-four on page 168. A Health Affairs survey indicates that the sickest 1% of the population in the United States uses 28% of the healthcare dollars. In this we have to assume that these are direct care funds, which can be defined as the total minus public health, research, and construction costs. This direct care cost totaled $1,077.1 billion in 1998. Estimating with this total, each patient of the 1% sickest Americans used $111,699 on average. The next percentile, according to the study, uses another 10% of the total, or an average of $39,892 per patient. The next three percentiles use 17%, which was $22,605 per patient on average. And 50% of the population used only 3% of the resources, or $239 per person. Some of these inexpensive patients are probably in fair to poor health but lack decent health insurance and access to the system. They then forgo medical services, primarily for reasons of cost. The 45% of Americans in between the expensive and inexpensive patients use 42% of the resources, or $3,719 per person on average.

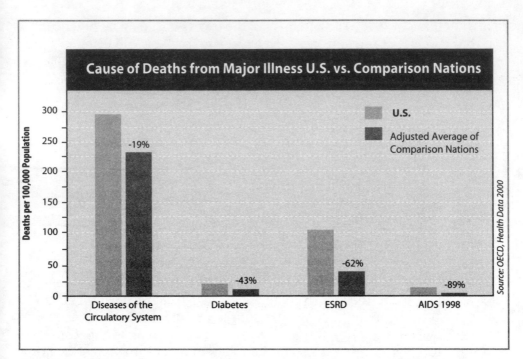

Figure Twenty-one

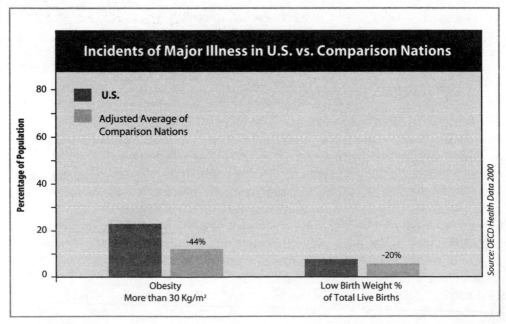

Figure Twenty-two

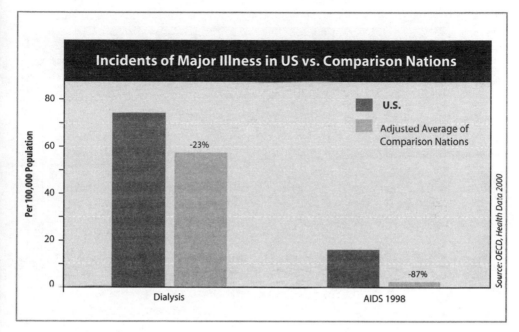

Figure Twenty-three

The OECD official population for the U.S. in 1998 was 270.3 million. Approximately 5.4 million Americans, the 2% who were theoretically the sickest, used about $75,366 on average and a total of $409 billion. The next 3% or 8,109,000 Americans used $22,605, each consuming $183 billion. America's most expensive and theoretically sickest patients, used $592 billion of the 1998 expenditure.

It is clear that 85 million Americans are uninsured or underinsured. It is also clear that uninsured persons are over represented in the 5,400,000 seriously ill citizens. *Consumer Reports* also demonstrated about 10% of Americans do not use medical services, insured or not, in a given year.[102] Refer to Figure Twenty-four on the next page. Nearly 70% of the chronically uninsured U.S. patients in poor health could not see a doctor when needed in the past year secondary to cost.[103] Many of these ill patients consume no healthcare costs and fall on the far right of Figure Twenty-four. But then they suffer a catastrophic illness and jump over the vast majority of Americans and join the most expensive patients on the far left of Figure Twenty-four. It is completely illogical for this wealthy democratic nation not to provide decent healthcare and insurance to the entire population.

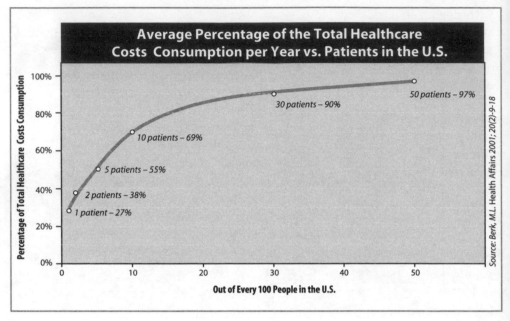

Figure Twenty-four

The study comparing insured and uninsured patients' use of preventive services found 10.3% of insured persons failed to obtain four key tests and 27.7 % of uninsured people also failed to obtain them, a factor of 2.7.[104]

Assuming these facts are correct, the uninsured people could be over-represented in the 2% of the seriously ill population. If 27% of the 43 million would not seek or could not get care over the years, then this has resulted in a large number of sick people who would likely not be sick in a universal care system. As they are also likely to be less well off financially, they are more vulnerable. When they get sick they become a cost to the system whether they can pay or not. In 1998, 27% of the 5.4 million very sick patients equals 1,462,000 people who become seriously ill because of our nation's failure to provide universal coverage, and cost our society over $110.1 billion in extra healthcare dollars. Similarly, uninsured citizens are over-represented in the next 3% who are not so sick. This calculates to 2,189,000 persons who are using $49.5 billion. The total cost of the sick and not so sick who should not be is $159.6 billion. And, this does not account for the underinsured.

Some will argue that the uninsured and underinsured are not taking care of themselves and lack individual responsibility. Earlier I have commented on the need for individual responsibility. This excess expense, however, is mostly not the patients' fault, but the blame should fall on this nation's health policy. America can afford to cover all people in this nation with decent healthcare from the beginning of their lives. The United States can prevent a large number, probably 3,651,000 people, from excess illnesses and costs by providing all people with decent healthcare and insurance.

Why do our nation's eyes remain closed to this major health injustice and tragedy? I believe most Americans fail to see the human suffering unless they are among the 3.65 million patients or their families. These Americans, who suffer needless illness, disability and premature death, are less than one out of every twenty uninsured and underinsured people. Most doctors remain silent, since these uninsured or underinsured patients are only fourteen patients per primary care doctor per year, or slightly more than one patient a month. And since doctors can block the access of these patients to their practice, they may rarely see these patients. For some people, including professionals, it is easy to dismiss these illnesses and look the other way.

There is a fourth proof of a very simple nature. Nations that enacted universal healthcare earlier in the 20th century enjoyed lower total healthcare costs in 1997. See Figure Twenty-five on page 170. And they will continue to do so, for they have been caring for their entire population for decades. This, I believe, is the fourth way that I can prove the United States has the highest healthcare costs from failure to provide universal coverage versus the comparison nations. In the United States we have sick people who would not be sick if they had access to decent healthcare from the beginning of their lives. Those nations that began to provide health insurance to greater than 99% of their population one-and-a-half or two generations ago, achieved lower overall costs in 1997 and 1998. America will not control medical costs until we give all of our people access to healthcare.

The existence of sick people who would not be sick if there were universal care may be the fundamental issue of the market-driven system. The market drive for the industry is contrary to providing coverage to the uninsured or the underinsured of society. Rather, the market drive is to deny primary care so that the underclass will get sick and become expensive patients for Medicare or others to pay for. The additional business for the healthcare industry was over $160 billion in 1998. This is a huge amount of money. And much of that business is due to the inadequacies of health care coverage and access, the degree of which is not seen in any other industrialized nation. This is a fundamental evil not tolerated in the comparison countries, the OECD nations as a whole, or nominally in any other signatory to the UN declaration of 1948. It is, hopefully, not the intention in the United States, but that is the effect. It is undeniable that this has to be rectified.

It is not necessary to explain every dollar Americans pay in the gap between our healthcare costs and the other large, industrialized, democratic

OECD countries. I know empirically that we have too many neglected sick patients in America, and many of these illnesses could have been prevented with a reasonable, equitable and just health system. Americans do not need to spend more for healthcare. Americans already spend plenty, but it is wasted on so many inefficiencies, greed and avoidable illnesses. There is much suffering and injustice in America, and many people are paying a heavy price. The costs, however, of not providing universal, comprehensive, quality healthcare are at least $160 billion. And that is not all of them.

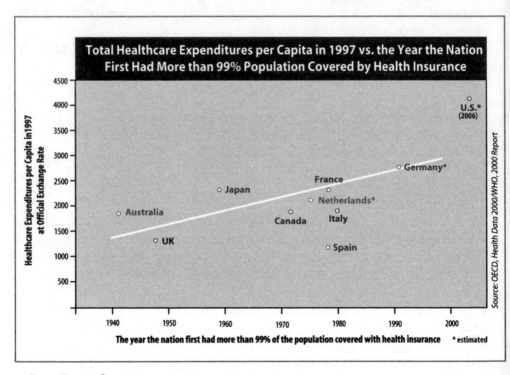

Figure Twenty-five

9: THE OTHER COSTS

"Rats and roaches live by the laws of supply and demand. It is the privilege of human beings to live under the laws of justice and mercy."

Wendell Berry

The lack of a universal care policy generates a cost not only in terms of direct healthcare expense for the great number of sick people, but also in terms of social and economic well being. The U.S. is a nation in which children are born into families without medical insurance or with too little of it. They receive significantly less pediatric care compared to fully insured families and every other family in the other wealthy industrialized nations. Families without the means try to find care in clinics, emergency rooms, and elsewhere. The same can be said for numerous working-age adults since one out of five lack health insurance in the United States. In reality, many children and adults have no primary care physician and fail to seek care until they sustain a serious, acute illness or suffer complications from untreated chronic diseases. If illnesses are not prevented or are left untreated they can progress, causing unfortunate consequences for these individuals. Some fail to obtain care and die prematurely. For others, their diseases are more advanced, leading to massive direct medical costs, and possibly even larger societal indirect costs. The deficiencies in the American health system manifest as a variety of problems, and the following are some examples.

Illegal Drugs, Legal Drugs, and Alcohol

While much of alcoholism and drug addiction originate with mental disease or family history, they are diseases that have preventive and therapeutic treatments. In a recent *Newsweek* report, drug addictions, direct and indirectly, cost society nearly $300 billion per year.[1] Forty-seven million Americans are addicted to cigarettes, fourteen million are addicted to alcohol and another 14 million people are addicted to illegal drugs. In New York State alone, 17%

of the entire federal allocation and state budget is spent on substance abuse related costs. This entails mainly enforcement and treatment. Only 1% of the 17% is spent on prevention or research.[2]

The $300 billion reported in Newsweek includes the cost of tobacco use. Implementing proven clinical smoking cessation interventions were estimated to cost $2,587 per life saved. This is far less than the indirect costs of continued smoking from lost productivity, early disability and premature death. Long-term smoking addiction causes more than just breathing problems.

As I stated in Chapter One, suicide attempts by elderly white men are often successful and not uncommon. Unfortunately, in one year, two of my patients were successful and another man was nearly successful. All three men had similar situations including advanced age, long histories of smoking and serious smoking-related health problems. Their advanced respiratory health problems led to feelings of hopelessness and marked depression. One man used a gun, another suffocated after drinking alcohol excessively and another overdosed on outdated sleeping pills. On the death certificates the coroner wrote suicide but I know they really died from chronic tobacco use and addiction.

About one in four Americans are currently smoking tobacco and face a lifelong addiction to a serious health hazard.[3] Many of these people will die prematurely from heart disease, cancer, emphysema or even suicide, as these aforementioned cases have demonstrated. Tobacco-related diseases are by far the most common cause of premature death in America, with diet and obesity being second, alcohol-related illnesses third, and accidental injuries fourth.[4]

Providing smoking cessation therapy to all smokers would be very cost effective in the big picture. Recent studies show that therapy costs approximately $2,600 for each life saved, but the insurance industry, including Medicare and Medicaid, fails to uniformly cover these services.

Universal access to medical care can treat smoking dependence.[5] If a smoker chooses to stop the habit, a two month supply of the prescription Zyban costs $150. If all of the smokers came to ask for cessation therapy in the same year, the cost would be $7 billion. For this one time $7 billion expenditure we could significantly reduce the use of tobacco and the mammoth direct and indirect costs weighing down our current health system. The U.S. easily spends far more money, estimated at $80 billion in 1999, for direct costs treating smoking-related illnesses including lung cancer, the most common cause of cancer death in this country.[6]

How much of the $300 billion in the *Newsweek* projection would be saved with universal healthcare is difficult to estimate. The war on illegal drugs is a popular cause with obvious merits, but it doesn't compare to the importance of a decent health system. Untreated drug or alcohol-related illness may touch your own life indirectly or directly someday.

It is well understood that addicts often turn to selling drugs or other crimes to maintain an adequate income to support their habit. In New York State, 21,000 out of 70,000 prison inmates are serving prison time for drug-related offenses. In this state, a conviction and prison term for selling two ounces of a controlled substance can equal the sentence of second-degree murder.[7] In other states the laws are not as severe, nevertheless, our nation's prisons are filled with drug offenders. Some estimate a one-year stay in a federal or state prison costs nearly $57,000 per inmate. Societal costs for drug abuse treatments are fourteen times less costly than incarceration. The Rand Corporation showed every dollar spent on substance abuse treatment saves taxpayers $7.46 in criminal justice and healthcare costs.[8] Addiction and crime are, in part, the result of not providing decent healthcare to every person in the U.S.

In the year 2000, according to the Justice Department, 12% of all black men between the ages of twenty and thirty-four were in prison.[9] Since the "war on drugs" intensified during the Reagan Administration, the number of incarcerated Americans and the length of illegal drug offenders' sentences have tripled while the proportion of inmates treated for substance abuse has more than halved during this same period.[10] In 1998, nearly one-half million people were in prison or jail for drug-related crimes. Most were users serving time for nonviolent crimes.[11] How many of these human beings would have their illnesses controlled after decent treatment for their addictions, either during or after their expensive prison stay? How many of these people will find gainful employment after their release? What are the chances they will remain "crime-free" or even "drug-free" without decent access to healthcare and treatment of their addictions? The real crime is that we have not provided all people in America access to decent medical care, and drug and alcohol treatments. How many crimes would have been prevented with a comprehensive national health program?

The war on drugs requires 100% medical access for those with addictions, not more prison terms. Alcohol and drug addiction are health conditions, and they are treatable. Without universal healthcare, people with the symptoms frequently can't seek help, nor can their family or friends find help for them.

The Tragic Ripples

When a stone is thrown into a quiet pond there are ripples that are easily seen and followed. However, when an uncovered and untreated patient is thrown into a dysfunctional health system, the ripples are not so easily detected nor followed. These ripples from a lack of universal healthcare in America can affect any of us and sometimes turn into tidal waves. A sad personal family story serves as a first illustration.

My sister married a family practitioner and moved to his lifelong rural community. They raised three great children in a loving home. Their oldest son was accepted at the Air Force Academy and actually flew an F-16. A few years ago, while driving home late one night from the Academy, he died in an automobile-equestrian accident. A horse accidentally escaped from an unlocked gate and wandered onto the rural highway. The police officer said my nephew had no chance of avoiding the accident when he came over the hill that night. Later we learned the horse's owner was an alcoholic and had been out drinking that same night while the horse was loose.

The funeral was powerful and sad. I remember the Air Force Cadets, our family and friends, so many who grieved with us. One could postulate whether this self-employed, farmer and horse owner, suffering from alcoholism, ever had decent access to medical care or substance abuse treatment. For our family, this man's probable untreated alcoholism caused more than just a ripple in our lives.

The pain, though, has not ended for my sister and our family. We were still suffering from my nephew's death when a second tragedy struck nearly one year later. One Sunday morning my sister and her husband were on a business vacation out of town and walking down a busy city street. An automobile driven by a known drug abuser accidentally jumped the curb and killed my brother-in-law instantly. Our family was, and is still, devastated. I remember the funeral service being filled with too many similarities. As the minister preached in the church about F-16 jets and God's power, we heard a jet fly randomly overhead, and the sound of the engine rumbled softly through the church. Another ripple in American healthcare has become a human tragedy of tidal wave proportions in our family.

There is possibly a profound meaning in these tragedies. I often wonder whether the alcoholic horse owner, who left the gate open while he succumbed to his disease, or the drug-abusing driver, who was possibly hallucinating when he accidentally killed my brother-in-law, ever had access to quality, affordable healthcare for their own health problems. Perhaps each ignored his physician's advice. Or possibly they were among those Americans who had no health insurance or lacked access to treatment when their diseases were in their early stages. Inaugurating universal care will not prevent all drug or alcohol addiction problems, but it will alleviate some. What mayhem do those who cannot get care cause to others and to our society at large, not to mention the huge economic costs?

There are other ripples. George, the carpenter from Chapter 1, represented some of the best qualities of the American worker. He was self-employed and hard working. George was also an independent and proud man. Without universal care throughout his life, it ended in the worst possible way. His family was rocked by the ripples. His sister frequently picked him up off the floor. Society picked up the check, a much larger check than it needed to be, all because this society choses not to provide decent health insurance to George, and to all people in our nation.

The Working Welfare Mother Syndrome is in itself another ripple. With one policy, government encourages women to enter into full employment with its attendant benefits to them and society. With another policy, government takes away their guaranteed health insurance, Medicaid, with all the portents of life disasters that can occur.

And then there was Lillian, who had an emergency amputation despite her attempt to obtain healthcare and her rejection by Medicaid years earlier. She had diabetes and cared for her ailing mother, but our society could not find the courage to provide universal health insurance for her. When her mother died, Lillian took on the added responsibility of caring for her mentally retarded sister. Now the question is, who will care for both of them now that Lillian is permanently disabled from a diabetic complication that was preventable. Our society cannot dodge the future bills and consequences of our failed system. For some the ripples fade away, but for others, the resultant tidal wave takes out entire families.

Mental Illness

Mental illness is an issue widely misunderstood by the public, with all of its associated stigmata. There are both psychological and physiological determinants of behavior; sorting them out for treatment is key! It requires a diagnosis and treatment, but that begins with decent access to healthcare and a personal physician.

A devastating weakness of the market-driven health system is an inability to respond to the cardinal point: mental illness is a human illness that needs a holistic approach. Despite the scientific evidence, insurance coverage by the private health insurance industry for mental health has steadily declined, forging wider inequalities between mentally and physically ill patients. Recent attempts in New York State to deliver parity in mental health have failed.[12]

The insurance industry lobby has effectively blocked any reasonable parity in mental health in New York State because of the potential of rising costs and more regulations. They will protect the industry, if possible, from undefined risks. But decent mental healthcare with parity for all people living in the United States will bring large indirect savings. The medical literature has shown that access to mental health services may decrease general medical costs, prevent absenteeism, lessen disability claims and reduce court and prison costs.[13]

Other states have passed parity laws with only minimal increases in overall healthcare premiums. Just recently, the federal government offered parity to federal employees, nine million of them, through their employer-sponsored, private health insurance plans. What took them so long? Nonetheless, well over 100 million Americans face disparity and unequal coverage with their health insurance when it comes to mental health, and drug or alcohol treatment.

One of my patients told me about her son Ben, who had schizophrenia, a chronic mental disorder, requiring long-term treatment and a trusting relationship. Ben had seen various doctors and had had treatments from his teenage years until the age of forty. I asked her, "What happened to your son, and how was he treated?"

She explained, "He was treated differently. Ben never had the same physician and had trouble obtaining help." She then went on to tell me about his last resort, a successful suicide attempt years earlier. She wanted to write about his story, but her pain was too great. I hope she will write Ben's story some day too; maybe other doctors would read it.

Prior to the 1960s, severe chronic mental disorders were treated with long-term psychiatric hospitalizations. The "wonder drug" discoveries of the last half-century have offered new hope to these patients and their families. These contributions by the pharmaceutical industry help to prove the stigma of mental illness is wrong. But the present system has not been developed for the continuous care of these patients with chronic health conditions. Many no longer require long-term hospital care as their symptoms are relieved with counseling and medications, but they still needed continuity of care by health professionals. This is an prime example of the need for comprehensive insurance in this nation; without it, the mentally ill are left to fend for themselves, and their symptoms soon return.

It seems that the market-driven system does not react to the patients' needs. Money has been saved, presumably, by closing mental hospitals. But if it has to be spent in building new prisons, what has this nation accomplished other than constructing a variety of expensive institutions? Access to consistent, quality mental healthcare is required to keep patients with mental health problems healthy. How do they get it without universal healthcare? If they don't receive proper treatment, the costs accrue to society by locking some of them up in well-fortified prisons. At present only Russia has a higher incarceration rate than the U.S. The yearly average prison incarceration costs in the U.S. are more than a Harvard education. The Los Angeles County Jail may be viewed as the largest mental health institution in the U.S. I think all Americans pay a steep price for untreated and under-treated mental disorders. Americans are treated differently if they have a mental disorder instead of a physical disorder. It surely would be more humane to treat and cover all mental illness with parity, and probably less expensive too.

Consider the fact that the median ages of mental illness onset are fifteen for anxiety, twenty-one for substance abuse disorder, and twenty-six for depressive disorders.[14] These disorders are also more common in segments of society that are disadvantaged such as the poor, less educated, or unemployed as well as unmarried populations. Anxiety is more common and chronic in women, while substance abuse is more common in men. Americans with mental disorders face more uninsurance and underinsurance issues compared to patients with physical disorders.

Tom, another patient with a chronic mental disorder, had just seen an alcohol treatment counselor but was referred to the emergency room for further treatment of his alcohol withdrawal. Tom told me he was required to bring in copies of his last four pay stubs before receiving treatment at the clinic weeks earlier. When I saw him in the ER his alcohol withdrawal symptoms had now progressed, requiring inpatient hospitalization. Why do we ask alcoholics to bring in copies of their pay stubs before treatment? Such absurd requests are not asked of asthmatic or diabetic patients.

I believe we need to treat mental and physical illness with parity and equal justice. Patients with mental, drug- and alcohol-related illnesses are discriminated against in the United States. Not only is it immoral and unjust, but it is also bad medicine.

Remember full-time employed Jennifer in Chapter One who attempted suicide after taking her sister's pills? Jennifer had symptoms of depression for many months and never sought help. This was partially because of her lack of insurance. She required treatment in the ICU and later a longer treatment in a psychiatric hospital. Obviously her care was expensive, but what if she had been successful? Untreated depression does kill people and hurts many others, including families and other loved ones. More ripples?

Suicide is the eighth most common cause of death in America and more common in people with drug or alcohol-related problems, a family history of suicide, previous suicide attempts or an untreated psychiatric illness.

Patients with mental illness need equality in healthcare. Does the private insurance industry remain more profitable by denying equal access, equal coverage and treatment for all mental disorders? When will the American people and our current health system end the stigma of mental illness and allow all sufferers access to decent mental health services?

The Aging of Society

Our society is aging as people are living longer, and that is good. According to the U.S. Census Bureau, the elderly population, age sixty-five and older, make up 13% of the entire population. The over eighty-five year age group accounts for the fastest growing segment of the American population.[15] However, with an aging population also comes more dependency and disability. One out of four people, age eighty-five and older, lives in a nursing home in the U.S., and 75% of all nursing home residents are women. Fifty-five percent of those who enter nursing homes will stay at least one year; 21% will remain five years or longer.[16] Nursing home care is expensive, averaging $41,000 per year (or $112 a day) in 1996.[17] Other figures show the costs to be even higher. In 1996, total national health expenditures for nursing facility care were $78.5 billion dollars, or 7.6% of total health expenditures for all services nationwide. That's $52,127 per patient per year.[18]

These nursing home costs, though, are primarily thrust onto the government and the patients themselves. Out-of-pocket costs average 31% in the U.S. for long-term care. Failure to prepare for the cost of nursing home care or other long-term care needs are a primary cause of impoverishment among the elderly, especially women.[19] The average widowed female lives six years longer than her male counterpart, but has less Social Security and retirement savings compared to her husband. Thus, elderly women in America succumb to poverty more commonly and for a longer duration.

In 1996, over 1.5 million patients lived in nearly 17,000 nursing facilities with a total of 1.8 million beds. The average U.S. nursing home has an 83% occupancy rate with 107 patient beds. Two-thirds of all nursing homes are for-profit. However, a recent study showed for-profit nursing homes having worse quality, 46.5% more citations for deficient care and 31% lower licensed nursing staff levels, compared to not-for-profit nursing homes.[20] This is yet another medical study demonstrating why the nation should dissolve investor-owned or for-profit institutions and providers in the direct care of patients.

In New York State the government, through Medicare, Medicaid, and the Veteran Administration, pays for over 90% of all nursing home costs. Some of the money comes through Medicaid after nursing home patients have turned over his or her home and other life's savings to the state.

Data comparing long-term care costs and nursing home utilization rates in other countries was very difficult to find. An older international study published in 1993 comparing long-term care in five countries, Australia, Canada, The Netherlands, Norway and United States, found many similarities for people living in nursing homes.[21] In four of the five countries, 4% to 5% of the elderly, age sixty-five and older, were living in nursing homes. Only 3% of the elderly in The Netherlands lived in nursing homes, nearly 40% less compared to the U.S. And a larger portion of The Netherlands population is elderly compared to the U.S. What is the difference between The Netherlands and the U.S. health systems?

One significant reason for The Netherlands' lower nursing home care utilization rate is the significant resources provided by their health system in providing formal home care services for 15% of their elderly population. Adult day care, home respite care and other support services allow families to continue to care for their elderly relatives outside of nursing homes. Since New York State taxpayers are already paying the vast majority of nursing home costs, why not expand publicly subsidized home care and allow many elderly patients to remain in their homes longer?

Obviously, for many Americans and New Yorkers, home health aides are simply not affordable, a situation I see frequently in my elderly patient practice. Carl, a veteran, was fully employed and working forty hours per week on his job. But he returned home to another full-time job, caring for his mother. His mother, also my patient, had advanced dementia. Luckily, Carl found adult day care services available for his mom while he was working. The problem for Carl was finding affordable home health aides on the weekends or at night. Carl described how his mother frequently wanders and hallucinates about relatives long gone. I asked him about a nursing home but he refused stating, "They'd have to drug her up, and then she'd be a vegetable. I'll deal with it as long as I can." He was probably right. My experience of over sixteen years would cause me to agree with him. Many patients with dementia are placed in nursing homes against their wishes and are later overmedicated in these "foreign" homes.

The stress on Carl was nearly unbearable. One time he said to me, "1999 was the worst year of my life! I wasn't under that much stress in Vietnam when they were shooting at me." Carl then explained to me how he had recently changed jobs, and his new employer did not offer prescription coverage. His high blood pressure and other medical problems required expensive medications. Instead of using his new employer-based health insurance, Carl remained on his old insurance that provided prescription coverage. "They screwed me earlier; now I'll screw them," he bluntly remarked. This is not the way our society should deal with such matters. When this man is overtaken by his stress and illness, the costs will easily rise exponentially for his mother's care, too.

I practice geriatric medicine, and, to me it is very likely that one-third of all U.S. nursing home patients, 500,000 people, could remain in their own homes, if only more home health services were affordable and available to them. U.S. families provide the majority of informal home care for their elderly loved ones already, well over 85%. I have seen many spouses or children over time become physically and emotionally overwhelmed trying to care for their loved one at home. I'm certain that most Americans would agree that patients remaining in their own homes or with their families leads to higher levels of patient care and satisfaction if affordable support were available.

Nursing home costs are approximately $41,000 per patient per year, with the majority of costs paid for by the government, nearly $37 billion in 1996. If a national health program provided home health aides to qualified patients with coverage up to $25,000 per year, there could be a substantial savings. With these affordable services for the patients and their families, I estimate one-half million Americans could be saved from "premature" nursing home care. Older persons prefer to be with their loved ones and friends. Since there is possibly an associated cost savings, why has this nation not proceeded to offer expanded home healthcare services for the elderly?

Hospice services are available to all terminally ill Americans, insured and uninsured. These patients can frequently remain home under hospice care with significant support for the patient and family. I remember the hospice nurse commenting, " Hospice is the first time Medicare actually meets the patient's entire needs." It is hard to put a value on this support; it is invaluable!

The Netherlands manages to provide home health services to 15% of their elderly population and have 40% fewer elderly patients in nursing homes. The Netherlands also has significantly lower overall healthcare costs compared to the United States. Instead, our market-driven system may find it more profitable to build large investor-owned chronic care facilities than to provide comprehensive long-term health insurance with adequate home health service coverage. Once again, the dichotomy: What is the object of the market drive? Is it what is best for the patient, or something else? Healthcare is too complex and the needs too fundamentally human to be left totally to free enterprise and price competition. There has to be an advocate for the patient and a system for all people. Instead we have lobbies that advocate for their special interests. In our nation we may have the most expensive lobby EVER!

The Cost of the Lobbies

The health industry lobby, with essentially false perceptions of the advantages of our market-driven system, has resisted this fundamental humanitarian concept in the United States. They spend millions on public propaganda and marketing techniques and possibly even more on politicians and their re-election campaigns. In the recent election of 2000, every candidate for Senate and nearly every candidate for the House of Representatives who spent the most money won their election.

The Medical Society of the State of New York (MSSNY) Political Action Committee (PAC) bragged recently how every candidate in the New York Senate whom they supported won their election. It was a "banner year in 2000." They only spent $830,000 on the state legislative candidates. Twenty-nine of thirty U.S. congressional candidates and 182 of 183 state legislature candidates supported by the PAC won election. An official stated, "The PAC activity is an important component of MSSNY's overall government relations strategy."[22]

The American Medical Association PAC donated more than $1.9 million directly to congressional candidates and spent an additional $1.8 million on commercials and direct mailings for the 2000 elections. Of these funds, 52% went to Republicans and 48% to Democrats. The AMA is one of the most politically potent lobbying groups in the nation's capital according to a spokesman for the Center for Responsive Politics, a nonpartisan research group. Someone said, "When the AMA talks, members of Congress listen." Maybe they should have said, "When someone gives enough money to Congress, they listen." American doctors are paid nearly twice the average of of their European counterparts and distort the political process to boot! Maybe we've met the enemy and he is us! Nearly two dozen other medical groups also contributed heavily to political candidates including the American Society of Anesthesiologists ($900,000), the American Optometric Association ($643,000), and the American Academy of Orthopedic Surgeons ($244,000).[23] The money, power and greed are so hard to let go of for the benefit of the patient.

I remember this phone call to my office one day. The caller was representing a U.S. congressman who was looking for community business leaders to serve on a congressional committee. I have spoken with many elected officials in our community about the sickness overwhelming our health system and its patients, and I thought they were looking for more of my input. I was initially surprised, honored and willing to serve, but then I asked some questions. The caller explained I could only serve on the committee if I gave them $300 to $500 for my services. My ego was deflated, for it was only a political fundraising phone call after all. I was willing to serve at no charge, but I was not willing to buy my committee seat.

A 1999 study suggested physician-lobbyists were focused on the bottom line and not on patient care. This study showed how most physician-lobbyists were focusing almost entirely on bottom-line issues such as Medicare reimbursement, managed-care reform and research funding. The same lobbyists frequently neglected such national public health issues as the uninsured, tobacco-control initiatives, abortion rights, and gun violence. "Luckily for physicians," the interviewed congressional aide stated, "their representatives are highly effective lobbyists and frequent visitors." The study's author stated, "I don't want to discount the importance of physician-lobbying on issues like reimbursement and managed care, but I don't think that excuses physicians from their responsibility to advocate for vulnerable patient populations." Another author stated, "Physicians have that obligation."[24] Physicians are not alone though when it comes to advocating for special interests rather than for the average American.

The pharmaceutical industry donated $19 million directly to candidates and national parties in the 2000 election. Unlike the doctors' PAC that nearly split donations between the two parties, the pharmaceutical industry heavily favored Republican candidates opposing the universal prescription coverage program as outlined by the Democratic presidential candidate. The industry feared a Medicare universal prescription coverage program would eventually lead to price controls and potentially lower profits. Two private drug companies each donated more money in 2000 than any other healthcare group or business in the entire nation. The drug industry spent another $50 million in television, newspaper, direct mail and radio advertisements through a pharmaceutical industry-backed group, Citizens for Better Medicare, and $10 million in similar fashion through the U.S. Chamber of Commerce.[25] The $80 million spent by the drug industry was the most expensive corporate effort in U.S. political history and it was twice the amount the tobacco industry spent in 1998 to defeat national settlements of government anti-tobacco lawsuits.

In addition to the huge amounts of money spent during this past national election, the PhRMA has spent approximately $360 million over the past decade for political contributions, lobbying, and advertising, all in the name of protecting their self-interests. The government has reciprocated by extending special tax breaks, drug-patent protections, direct-to-consumer advertising and generous basic governmental research support for the industry.[26] During this same period the sick patients and the elderly in the U.S. have also seen higher drug prices, medical inflation, and possible quality concerns. As mentioned earlier, 16% of all the drugs approved in the year 1997 have been removed from this nation's and other nations' markets because of safety issues.[27]

The drug industry and their lobby obviously have taken their message to the public and Congress in times of need. But now I am seeing their lobbying efforts focus directly on the doctor too.

A drug representative recently told me about his new product on the market and the potential benefits. He also mentioned how the drug has been used in Canada for "a long time," but he "was not supposed to tell" me that. During this particular encounter, the drug representative also commented, "The reason for the high costs of healthcare in this country is the government. The second problem is people think healthcare is a right, and it is not. And then people think medical care is free." He tried to explain how it was the government's fault that drugs take so long to get developed in this country. "The average time from application until approval has gone from seven to over twelve years in the U.S.," he claimed. He even added the standard PhRMA line that it costs $500 million on average for R&D on each drug approved in the U.S. I knew his facts were inaccurate and misleading. Of course he was quoting a PhRMA study from 1991 that has never been reproduced. I recently read about a report from a group called Public Citizen questioning the PhRMA 1991 claim. Public Citizen estimated the costs, at $110 million per new drug developed since the previous PhRMA study includes tax-deductible expenses, over-estimates of risks and minimizes the public's contributions to medical research.[28]

Unfortunately, I was already behind in my office hours. Otherwise I would have responded to him. It is a complex issue obviously, and so easy to point the finger at everyone else. Blame the government. Blame the patients. Blame the basic human rights tenet that grants access to healthcare as a basic right in nearly all other democratic countries of the world except ours. Obviously new medications are expensive to develop regardless of whether the actual average cost is $110 million or $500 million. That is one of the many reasons why our nation needs to develop new drugs that truly make a real difference in the care of the patient.

After the drug representative left my office, I telephoned the FDA. I was told the average time of a new drug application (NDA) until approval by the FDA has been reduced from twenty-two months to twelve months in recent years, thanks to changes made by Congress in 1997.[29]

For now, though, it appears to me the drug industry may not only be taking its product messages to the doctors, but also to their "lobby" party line. As I have said before, the industry is good at what it does, marketing their products and lobbying their own self-interests.

There are powerful lobby groups with special interests. The HMOs and other health service providers' direct donations to political campaigns grew to $5.8 million in the 2000 election.[30] In Massachusetts alone, during the 2000 elections, the "not-for-profit" HMOs spent over $5 million dollars attacking a ballot initiative, Number Five, calling for universal health insurance in the state. The HMOs outspent the supporters of this initiative a hundred fold. The ballot initiative called for universal insurance with a cap placed on insurance administrative costs at 10%, and a ban on "for-profit" hospitals and insurance companies. The ballot initiative was successfully defeated by the HMO industry, but by a very narrow margin. Unfortunately, since the defeat of this initiative, news reports have documented more instances of Massachusetts emergency room overcrowding, ambulance drive-bys, rising costs and greater numbers of uninsured people.

The insurance industry is big business in other states too, including New York State, accounting for $90 billion per year. To maintain their powerful control and self-interests, the industry maintains large numbers of lobbyists in Albany, the state capital. According to a study by the New York Public Interest Research Group, 115 insurance industry interests hired 83 lobbying firms in 1997 at a cost of $6 million to lobby in the state capital. For the decade prior to the year 2000, only one person had been chairman of the NY State Senate Insurance Committee. As one insurance lobbyist stated, "Anybody who doesn't pay attention to… is an idiot." The lobby need only apply significant and effective force on certain individuals to control an entire industry.[31]

In 1993, special interest groups devastated the Clinton health plan. The multiple lobbies, along with "Harry and Louise" commercials, attacked other nations providing universal coverage as inadequate and inferior to the U.S. They maintained that doctors in these countries were poorly paid and inept, and that most new drugs were not developed outside the U.S. The lobbies generated tremendous fear, portraying the Clinton plan as a bureaucratic monster. It was, they said, a healthcare plan that would restrict a patient's choice of doctor or hospital and would ration needed care to millions of patients. The lobbies were successful and the plan was defeated, leaving most elected officials fearful of any major overhaul of the present U.S. healthcare system and fearful of not being reelected should they oppose the lobby. But the reality is that there are long waiting lines in the United States for the underclass and care is being rationed by not providing care to all. What kind of healthcare system do most Americans face today in the year 2001? I believe that the fears of the Clinton plan so many lobbies vigorously promoted are what millions of Americans face today, and we still leave one out of seven people without any health insurance. The fears promulgated by the lobbyists include, uncontrolled medical inflation, rationing, worsening services, litigation, bureaucracy nightmares, and loss of freedom in choosing a provider and hospital. The lobby is good at what it does; otherwise the United States would have had a national health program for all people decades ago and a healthier society today. "The societal costs of licensing lawyers to distort and conceal are especially great when they represent large and powerful organizations with the capacity to cause disease, death, or mis-information," an author once commented about another large U.S. industry.[32] Could the same be said of the U.S. healthcare lobby?

The general opinion seems to be that the cost of implementing any national health program would be too high. However, if our society fails to enact a universal national health program, health costs will spiral ever higher, and necessary care will continue to be denied to many Americans.

Taxes

What probably instills fear in most Americans is the possibility of higher taxes. If we include public employees' health insurance premiums covered by their employer, 51% of the 1998 total healthcare expenditures came from public funds.[33] Where do the tax dollars come from that pay for healthcare services in this nation? Most working Americans potentially faced the Medicare tax of 2.9% split equally between the employee and the employer costing $213 billion in 1998.[34] As of March 2000, New York State's total revenues were $38.2 billion with personal income taxes accounting for $22.4 billion. New York State medical expenditures were $6.2 billion for Medicaid (16.3% of total revenues) and $3.0 billion for New York State employees (7.8% of total revenues) or 24.1% of all tax dollars for New York State residents.[35] Chautauqua County, where I reside, has 140,000 people, who paid county property taxes totaling $37 million in 2000. The Medicaid contribution was $19.5 million (52.7%) and $2.8 million (7.6%) for county employees health benefits or 60.3% of our total county taxes. The state must also contribute 25% and the federal government another 50% of the total cost of Medicaid. Total Medicaid expenditures were $136 million, nearly $1,000 for every single person living in our county. Even our local school taxes provide health insurance for the public teachers and employees at $1.32 million or 16.4% of taxes. Jamestown, the largest city in Chautauqua County, recently levied a $2 million tax rate increase with over one-half of the increase secondary to rising city employee health insurance costs, nearly 13% of the total city budget.[36]

In 1998, the average New York State resident paid $4,687 in total health expenditures ($85.8 billion total) with $27 billion in Medicaid and $18.7 in Medicare.[37] I estimate another $3 billion was spent for public employees and another $6.5 billion for government programs such as the VA, Champus, worker's compensation and other programs. In reality, New Yorkers paid for nearly two-thirds of their healthcare with tax dollars. And that does not include all of the tax exemptions for employers and individuals who pay for private insurance. Then, the percentages would be even higher.

When I examined the medical expenditures of the other forty-nine states, it appeared that states with higher percentages of public total funding costs in general also had greater per capita healthcare overall costs.[38] Why do these public versus private funding differences among the states differ from my findings in the comparison nations versus the entire United States? I believe the answer lies in what happens after the taxes are collected. In the United States public funds collected through taxes and marked for healthcare services are frequently left to the control and management of the private insurance industry, many of which are for-profit. In the comparison nations, their programs are publicly financed and much more likely to be publicly administered. And if private insurance companies administer the program, they are essentially not-for-profit. These are significant differences between the U.S. and the comparison nations.

I frequently hear our elected officials at all levels of government ask for more private health insurance participation, many for-profit, to manage the public's dollars and health insurance programs. In New York State, essentially all Medicaid patients will be forced to enroll in private HMO insurance programs. It is a major windfall for the private insurance industry and will fail to control costs and medical inflation long term.

The insurance industry has perfected the ability to delay provider payments or to deny claims, thus accruing over one billion dollars each year in interest. And if they find no easy profits, they drop participation and dump the patients back onto the original government programs. The HMO industry is doing precisely these things to the American people. HMOs are dropping Medicare patients in droves, while at the same time, asking for more money from government.

These numbers are probably overwhelming to the average person and perhaps even too confusing for our leaders in government who have access to this information. Remember, your tax dollars already pay 51% of all healthcare dollars in this country and two-thirds of all costs in New York State. And yet, there is such resistance in this country to having universal care with a single-payer mechanism for a funding source. Why? Maybe we would really know how much it actually cost if we had one simple funding system. Maybe we would bring costs under control with the best care available for all, not just the well off and the well insured.

America does not have the best healthcare system in the world, and we are not getting full value for our money. The vast majority of large democratic OECD countries have better health outcomes and greater satisfaction. Many of the countries support primary care based systems and still provide patients the freedom to choose their doctor. These same countries insist on universal coverage for all people providing physical, mental and dental health services while still costing less in out-of-pocket expenses, healthcare taxes, and overall health expenditures compared to the U.S.

I believe even basic health care that is provided to all people in the United States will deliver a healthier patient and society when compared to our current dysfunctional, market-driven system. And patients with combined Medicare and Medicaid services do receive more than just basic healthcare. See Figure Eighteen. Comprehensive publicly funded and publicly administered health programs can deliver quality medical care to the American people. The health insurance industry and its lobbies, along with many politicians, have the public fooled into thinking their government is inefficient at operating a decent health insurance program.

How do the American people defeat the lobby? By developing a plan that covers all human beings comprehensively, compassionately, justly and cost-effectively, which is not provided by the current MSA proposals or tax-incentives being proposed. The MSA program the United States could enact is "Medicare Services for All." But we need more than just a national health program.

In the final chapter I present my treatment plan for all Americans. My prescription offers no simple pills to take and the recovery will take time. But this nation's health system can overcome the sickness of profits over patients.

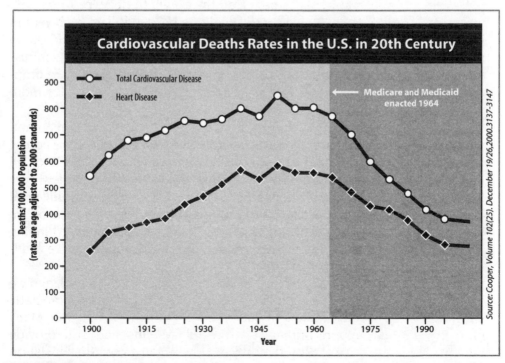

Figure Eighteen

10: THE TREATMENT

"Do not allow thirst for profit, ambition for renown, and admiration to interfere with my profession for these are the enemies of truth and can lead me astray in the great task of attending to the welfare of your creatures."

Prayer of Maimonides c1190 AD

Within the American healthcare system there are supposed to be better-equipped, better-managed, and better-staffed hospitals per million people than most other nations. For those people in this country who have high-quality, comprehensive health insurance, the system rates well in terms of patient satisfaction. The ratings are high for our medical schools, our teaching and our research. The government institutions of the National Institutes for Health (NIH) and the Center for Disease Control (CDC) are possibly the best in the world. The pharmaceutical industry is part of the multi-national industry of famous corporations, and produces miracle drugs for the patients of the world. Yet, doctors leave their profession in disgust, and nurses do the same.

Doctors see daily the patients who can't afford to care for themselves. They try, as I do, only to become frustrated with the system. They see the patients cutting their pills in half, patients saying that they can't have a needed operation because they can't pay, people with illnesses that could have been prevented. Doctors are deluged with paperwork from the multiple-payer bureaucracies who push it out of their offices onto them as claimants. They are harassed by HMO and insurance company reviewers and often insulted by their requests. There is a deep feeling of loss of autonomy and professionalism.[1] Their cash flows are stressed by the slowness of payments as insurance companies seem to keep their rivers of cash in a float (i.e. earning interest), as long as they can. They are always conscious of the plaintiff lawyers who advertise their victorious settlements in ever-increasing amounts. Their own professional associates offer them appeals to greed;

"The system will never change. You should make as much money as you can." Greed may be the real concern. So I ask again, what has happened to the profession? Why do some practitioners too often wonder if they like being doctors? Some feel they are no longer as respected as doctors once were.

For hospital workers, executives and medical staff, the same issues apply. The paperwork from the insurance companies and HMOs is overwhelming. The insurance industry bureaucracy is hostile. Cash flow is always a problem; the budget is even worse, particularly for public hospitals that are required to take the really sick people who come to them when there is no other source of care.

It is a reality in the American system that patients are objects of necessary discrimination and most people in healthcare don't like to discriminate between people who need care. I believe only a few are unfeeling and calloused and they probably don't belong in healthcare. Doctors, nurses and other health professionals almost universally want to make patients well, to prevent illness or to relieve their patients' discomfort.

The United States has about 85 million people; or possibly 33 million households, with no or inadequate insurance. By an OECD survey, 55% of American households do not have adequate coverage by OECD standards.[2] This includes those who in their insurance or HMO plans are prohibited from receiving various treatments or manipulated to go to certain clinics, physicians or hospitals. The very important relationship with their personal physician is broken. The most often cited reason for a change in physicians is a requirement by an insurance program. American doctors see this almost daily and most are sensitive to it.

In the name of the market-driven system which supposedly bestows liberty and great benefits to all Americans unavailable in other nations, the industry struggles to control public opinion. The industry lobbies also exert their powerful influence on members of Congress, on the Department of Health and Human Services, on leaders of the political parties and on the White House. The lobby loudly criticizes other nations' universal health systems while ignoring the tragedy in our own faltering system.

Instead of a national health program providing universal care to all people, America has attempted a myriad of incremental programs: Medicare, Medicaid, commercial insurance, HMOs, self-insurance, MSAs, Worker's Compensation, Child Health and Family Health Plus, VA, etc. Americans always hear the call for "market forces." We delay the enactment of a truly universal national health policy with a mythology of a "Patient's Bill of Rights" based on the right to sue insurance companies and HMOs. I believe this again demonstrates the concept of incremental reform. It seems the lobby's strategy is to prevent comprehensive reform in the United States that would bring quality, affordable, accessible healthcare to all people and public accountability to the entire industry. Small incremental programs can be manipulated to create an illusion of progress.

Unfortunately, this incremental reform has created an awful reality for some Americans. Many are still falling through major cracks in a broken system. They suffer ill health, early disability, and premature death that could have been avoided with any decent universal system. As individuals and a nation, we do have the ability to change and improve our overall health. It will take a combined approach of individual responsibility and a workable national healthcare program that takes into account the realities of peoples' lives and needs.

Individual Responsibility

We should first focus on individual health and responsibility. Clearly, science and common sense demonstrate the importance of regular exercise, eating properly, not smoking, limited alcohol use if any, avoiding illicit drugs, using seatbelts, "abstinence" or "safe sex" and other obvious examples. We are, on the other hand, only human beings who stumble along life's journey and can fall from the better path. Some people eat the wrong foods, smoke too much, drink too much, abuse drugs, work too hard, and so on, but recovery is possible.

I remember Trent in the emergency room reeking of alcohol, bleeding profusely from just about every orifice, and swearing at everyone that tried to help him. Later, he was hallucinating and shaking terribly from alcohol withdrawal. We also found liver disease, emphysema and cancer. I didn't think that he would survive these illnesesses or change his ways. Nearly seven years later, however, Trent is one of my favorite patients. He changed his life. He has stopped smoking and drinking alcohol, infrequently misses appointments and takes his medications faithfully. Trent even watches his diet and exercises. He loves life. None of us expected that this man could achieve such an amazing recovery! He demonstrates to me the remarkable ability of the human being to adapt and change. People are able to overcome their addictions, illnesses, and other "bad habits," especially if they have the support they need, including a loving family, the will to live, and some luck. I must add, Trent also had comprehensive health insurance which gave him access to affordable, quality healthcare.

How much can individuals change? My sister is another example. She was always a lot of fun to be around, and still is. When we were young, I remember her hiding vegetables from Grandma's dinners under a napkin at the dinner table or even in a nearby plant. She was brilliant; she could get out of eating any of those "yucky" vegetables. Did she exercise? No way, not my sister. She smoked and probably drank her fair share of alcohol in college. She eventually overcame the tobacco addiction and stopped alcohol use. She became a vegetarian, but she still hated vegetables. Then her weight climbed to dangerous levels.

Something changed in her life, a health scare or a wake-up call. Only she knows, but it demonstrates the amazing recovery humans can make in their lives. Now a true vegetarian, she loves her organic foods, exercises hours per day and looks and feels great. She is now the best athlete in our family, and has even trained for a triathlon.

People are making differences in their health now and for the future. These stories are important because optimal health and disease prevention cannot be reached without individuals accepting responsibility for their health. Hopefully, responsible individuals will serve as role models, leading others to also accept their individual responsibility and not fall so far into ill health. Many individuals have the strength and courage to climb out of their predicament. They are the inspirations. This individualism is not something that can be programmed into a society or proselytized successfully. Healthcare, however, goes beyond individual responsibility.

Access for All

I believe all people need access to a doctor in whom they have confidence and trust. Everyone wants a doctor who places his or her patient's health needs first, instead of personal income or practice profit margins. Everyone needs a personal physician who educates, provides guidance, counsels, makes diagnoses and provides treatment. Does this physician have to be a "primary care provider" who practices in fields of family practice, Internal medicine, pediatrics, or obstetrics and gynecology? No, I think not. Some patients need access to many doctors or may even need other specialists as their primary physician.

Everyone deserves treatment without regard to "ability to pay" or other prejudices. The American discrimination by healthcare providers between rich and poor, young and old, white and non-white, male and female must end. Our system must provide the best care humanly possible to every individual, and insist that each patient be treated as he would want himself or family members treated. Maybe that is a new "Golden Rule" of healthcare.

Freedom of Choice

Patients also need and deserve the freedom to choose their doctors, whether for primary care or specialist treatment and to choose their hospital, nursing home, other treatment facilities and pharmacy. Right now the healthcare underclass of Americans, and a good many others, don't have these freedoms. If they are established, these new freedoms will build social trust, and improve the quality of care and patient satisfaction. Competition in healthcare cannot be about price and market shares. But there should be competition based on quality and service to patients. To allow competitive forces to improve these factors, patients must have access to any licensed provider of their choice. Such access requires a national health program and universal coverage.

Universal Health Insurance

If the stories I have told fail to convince anyone that all Americans need universal coverage and access, then remember there are well over 100 different medical studies which have documented better overall healthcare and outcomes for insured versus uninsured patients. If this is not convincing, then remember the excessive cost of $160 billion per year for Americans needlessly sick from previously untreated and uncovered illnesses. If that is not convincing, then add the indirect societal costs and all the human tragedy.

This national health program must provide universal insurance that is comprehensive, portable, non-discriminating, high quality, and affordable to all people. It must cover all people regardless of their ability to pay, whether in (or out) of the hospital. It must be health insurance that covers the majority of costs related to medical, mental, dental, prescription, and long-term healthcare needs. Out-of-pocket costs should be minimized as much as possible and ideally limited to less than 10% of total income for an individual or family. In 1998, Americans spent $199.5 billion out-of-pocket, and much of that came from the uninsured or underinsured people. Many elderly, even with Medicare, now spend over 25% of their income on healthcare. And as you have seen, the uninsured can spend their entire life savings and high percentages of their current income for needed care. By "quality insurance" I mean that it must be comprehensive by covering over 90% of the costs, providing patient- and caregiver-friendly service and eliminating the waste inherent in the multiple-payer and HMO bureaucracies.

Undertaking this insurance program would vest all Americans with healthcare as a right. Our law generally grants that all persons are equal before it. This should become the case in healthcare as well. Do Americans really want their doctors treating them differently because of the insurance they carry (if any) or the amount of money they have in their pocket? When I say patients should be treated equally, I don't mean physicians should prescribe the same dose of medicine to every single patient. I mean patients should be treated according to their medical problems and health conditions and not according to their bank accounts or insurance plan. All

Americans deserve the best possible care from their physician, nurse, hospital or therapist regardless of their status or plight in life.

The New York State Hospital Bill of Rights states all patients have the right to receive medical treatment without discrimination as to race, sex, color, national origin, disability, sexual orientation or source of payment. But why do we grant this right only in the hospital? What happens before and after the hospital? Why the difference in location? Besides, most medical care is delivered outside of hospitals.

Frequently in the United States, when new patients call for a doctor's appointment, the first question the patient hears is, "What's your insurance?" Sometimes the doctor's office fails to even ask for a name. Some Americans get an appointment, and some do not. Sometimes the questions are even harder to swallow, such as, "Do you have the money to pay?" Americans are frequently victims of discrimination in healthcare simply because of their inability to pay.

Even if there is no discrimination by healthcare professionals in the hospital or emergency room, what happens to the patients next? Are patients not treated differently once they leave the hospital? Frequently patients facing high out-of-pocket costs or inadequate insurance will not fill their necessary prescriptions or go for follow-up appointments. Some physicians examine and treat hospitalized patients and then later refuse these same patients return appointments simply because of the patient's lack of money or "well-paying" insurance. Patients in the United States are treated differently because of their inability to pay outside the hospital, an experience well known by too many Americans. Furthermore, if hospitals are for-profit or face financial pressures, they sometimes discriminate against patients by type of insurance or ability to pay. These discriminatory practices only lead to a worsening of the patient's overall health.

There is strong evidence that the public supports universal healthcare as a basic human right. The late Cardinal Joseph Bernardin from Chicago, Illinois, stated, "Healthcare is an essential safeguard of human life and dignity and there is an obligation of society to ensure that every person be able to realize this fundamental right."[3] In 1999, a referendum was placed before the voters that called for an amendment to the Illinois State Constitution to enact a plan that permits everyone in that state to obtain decent healthcare on a regular basis. Called "The Bernardin Amendment," voters approved and passed the amendment by 83% in Cook County, which includes Chicago, Illinois, and 71% of the entire state of Illinois.

In a 1999 NBC News/ *Wall Street Journal* poll, 67% of Americans thought the Federal Government should guarantee health insurance coverage for every American.[4] I believe most Americans would support an "improved"

Medicare-based national health program for all people if they were fully informed.

As a practicing doctor, citizen, father, husband and patient, I believe that all people have the right to quality healthcare in this nation. This nation is founded on the principles of life, liberty and the pursuit of happiness. Life requires decent access to medical care. Liberty means freedom to choose your doctor, hospital or other provider, and freedom to change jobs, travel, retire, move, marry, or seek help. Pursuit of happiness is difficult for those who are overcome by illness or are chronically sick. Do you remember the last time you really felt sick? What if you could not afford healthcare or were afraid to seek help?

A National Healthcare Program

The specifics of my recommendations are as follows:

1. Establish a National Health Program (NHP) guaranteeing the right to quality healthcare for all people living in the U.S. and provide every person comprehensive health insurance with a single-payer mechanism. Extend Medicare as a NHP to the entire population with an improved structure eliminating most co-payments and high deductibles, and expand prescription coverage to cover at least 90% of the drug costs. Out-of-pocket health costs should not exceed 10% of any individual's or family's total income.

2. Phase out all for-profit or investor-owned provider and insurance organizations with a one-time fair buyout of all such organizations. Return HMOs to their former role of not-for-profit, providing comprehensive services to their patients.

3. Provide basic dental care for every person living in the United States.

4. Establish a permanent national commission to define global budgeting for hospitals; to consider fixed fees for pharmacists; to negotiate fees with physicians, dentists, and other licensed providers, paying them according to their specialty and time spent with patients; and to set maximum prices for pharmaceuticals, while allowing manufacturers a significant profit in return for the risks they take.

5. Fund the National Health Program with a simplified and progressive taxation mechanism.

6. Provide for retraining of workers who are displaced from insurance companies by the enactment of a NHP and increase the number and possible earnings of nurses, home health aides, therapists, social workers and others.

7. Provide for long-term care for all patients suffering chronic disabling illnesses, with emphasis on extending home health services and support for their families and communities.

8. Establish that the patient-physician's decisions are final. Allow patients the right to second opinions. Continue or upgrade policies under which providers should maintain competency, board recertification and continuing medical education requirements.

9. Focus the nation's medical research spending on diseases that cause significant premature death and disability such as tobacco addiction, obesity, diabetes, accidents, tuberculosis, diarrheal illness, drug addiction and mental illness.[5] Increase clinical research, evaluating new therapies and medications against current standard treatments. Constantly seek to improve the quality of existing therapies and treatments.

10. Provide the payment of the education costs for students who are accepted into the nation's medical and dental schools.

11. Establish a voluntary patient data bank of personal medical records maintained by the patient's primary care physician with assured confidentiality. Allow for instant access by emergency providers in medical emergencies with all other releases requiring the patient's consent. Encourage the general use of electronic medical records.

12. Enact malpractice reform providing alternative dispute resolution, administrative mediation, and a no-fault compensation system for medical injuries.

The Start-Up Costs

Foremost in the opposition to such a plan is the question of cost. Part of the answer is obvious in Chapter Eight. The American people already spend 58% more than the weighted average of the comparison nations for healthcare. Those who have access are likely no better off than individually responsible, well cared for Europeans. As a nation America's health delivery system is a disgrace. But, despite the overall mediocre results, what is the point of argument to people who can afford it? Namely, it is a system wasteful beyond belief and manipulated by a lobby focused on providing the highest profits for their self-interests and investors, and mammoth cash flows to companies that should not exist or not be involved in healthcare. The system is also paying for an extremely large number of sick people who would not be sick under any decent universal healthcare system. This is a matter of social injustice of the first magnitude, "most shocking and inhumane," as Dr. Martin Luther King eloquently stated.

The real issue should be whether discrimination and lack of access to decent healthcare are tolerable in a democracy. Sadly, the ultimate issue will be the cost in shifting from a dysfunctional and fragmented system to a National Health Program that establishes universal quality care and mitigates private exploitation. The following is an economic analysis, assuming the adoption of a National Health Program, as recommended above:

In Chapter Eight, the cost of American healthcare versus the weighted average of the nine comparison nations showed various excesses in 1998, some of which could be reduced by a national policy. These were:

Excess marketing costs in pharmaceuticals	$10.9 billion
American pricing of pharmaceuticals	$13.7 billion
Excess cost of multi- payer insurance	$43.9 billion
Excess administrative cost	$46.5 billion
Malpractice insurance/defensive medicine	$31.9 billion

In a referenced study, the uninsured citizens in the U.S. are estimated to receive about 60% of medical services compared to the well-insured citizens.[6] This includes the very expensive treatments, which I have described, and other treatments for which they may or may not pay. The aggregate of the medical services received in 1998 by all Americans was:[7]

Hospital revenue	$383 billion
Physicians revenue	229
Home and nursing home care	117
Pharmaceuticals	122
Other professional services	67
Optometry	16
Other services	32
Total	$966 billion

The study does not include the 42 million underinsured persons, according to the calculations in Chapter Two and the 63 million whom the OECD indicates are not fully insured. They are subject to the various limitations imposed by insurance companies and HMOs. An assumption is necessary: the underinsured described in Chapter Two receive 80% of the amount of health services compared to the fully insured. The remaining people indicated by the OECD to be less than fully covered, receive 95% of the services compared to those who are fully insured.

Given the defined total direct healthcare expense of $966 billion, the 122 million people fully insured would have used an average of $4,206 per capita. The 63 million with questionable insurance would have used $3,992 per capita by the above assumption. The 42 million underinsured citizens would have used $3,332 per capita and the 43 million uninsured citizens would have received $1,633 per capita. The shortfall of the underinsured was $874 each or $36.7 billion for the 42 million and $13.4 billion or $214 each for the 63 million identified by the OECD. The shortfall of uninsured Americans was $1,682 each, or $72.3 billion. This means that if America had changed completely to the new policy in 1998, uninsured and underinsured persons could have claimed $122.4 billion in new services by these assumptions. That would be a significant increase, even though the new policy would eventually save $160 billion in excess spending for sick, uncovered people under our sick system.

However, with a single-payer system and the National Health Program boldly applied, there will be multiple near-term savings. Reversing the excess underwriting margins and profits of the multi-payer insurance companies yields $43.9 billion; another $46.5 billion comes from providers' excessive administrative costs. By pushing the plaintiff bar out of medicine, another $22.9 billion could be saved by making defensive medicine unnecessary. Another $10.9 billion can be saved in pharmaceutical industry marketing. This is an offset of $124.4 billion.

Surveys indicate that approximately 10% of insured adult Americans do not utilize health services in a given year.[8] Granting healthcare as a human right to the previously uninsured and underinsured citizens will not guarantee that all of these previously untreated or under-treated patients will utilize the newly formed system. A 90% utilization of $122.4 billion in new services would total $110.2 billion. This could be considered "a wash" in start-up costs with a $12.2 billion or a 11% margin of error. There could be some delay in realizing the savings if the program is not fully implemented.

Enacting a National Healthcare Program under an improved universal Medicare for all Americans would significantly reduce medical inflation and total health expenditures to nearly 12.5% of GDP over a five year period. Further savings will immediately accumulate with reduced indirect societal costs.

The pharmaceutical industry should benefit with higher sales, even at negotiated prices, as all Americans should be able to fill their prescriptions. A net savings for society is also possible with less marketing costs expressed in lower prices. Volume could increase 20% as all Americans have full access to healthcare and more likely fill their prescriptions. High profitability in this industry would be maintained.[9]

There will be a loud shout from the lobby claiming the system will be overwhelmed with patients taking advantage of a "free" system. Those who maintain this narrow-minded view forget that the vast majority of Americans have better things to do than to run to the doctor or dentist for trivial matters on a frequent basis. Most people seek care when they have symptoms, are injured or in need of preventive health services. The lobby forgets or overlooks the reason for the profession of medicine in the first place, to care for patients. When they claim that "free care" will overwhelm the system, they also seem to be the same voices that cry out against rationing in other nations' systems. How ironic for a lobby to criticize rationing in other nations, while imposing rationing in America by providing the highest prices for medical care in the world, and no guaranteed universal care system in place. Some claim "free care" may also lead to excessive tests and treatments.

Current over-testing and over-utilization rates by some Americans are more likely related to our system's failure to provide a decent national health program for all people instead of the "free care." Many Americans lack access to a personal physician who can solve their health problems, answer their questions or alleviate their fears the majority of the time. Doctors also fear "making mistakes" or "messing up" and malpractice actions. Treating providers frequently lack previous patient information and test results, leading to even more repeated tests and procedures. Many providers make more money performing more tests and services on patients, which may not be clinically necessary. As the wealthiest nation in the world, we also spend more money on research developing new technologies and medications that frequently are expensive. In the end, regardless of the system, it will still be the providers' responsibility, doctors, dentists, therapists and others, to not over-treat or over-test the patient. As health professionals, we also have a responsibility to all patients not to under-treat or under-test them either. It is too easy to blame the patient, for a truly just and fair system would demand and expect much greater actions of its healthcare providers.

The Financing

Obviously Americans are not getting what they paid for when one considers our overall healthcare results and costs. Our healthcare costs are hidden in sales taxes, taxes on tobacco and alcohol, state and local income taxes on individuals and businesses, Medicare employer and employee taxes, and real estate taxes. Presently the Medicare tax rate is specific, and the federal income tax, business taxes and excise taxes are a source of all types of health expenditures. Taxes for healthcare extend to the states, counties, cities and towns which have public health departments, mandatory Medicaid expenses, public medical institutions and public assistance for individuals. Our healthcare costs are also buried in insurance premiums for health, automobile, homeowner's, malpractice, life, disability policies, and worker's compensation. Americans pay the third highest out-of-pocket costs in the world as a percentage of total healthcare costs.[10]

Most Americans are aware that hospitals, doctors, and others inflate their charges for services to cover the costs of caring for people who cannot pay. The question of what percentage of the services received by uninsured citizens are actually paid for requires speculation. The average American per diem room charge is much higher than in the comparison nations. The use of resources by uninsured citizens totals $92.2 billion according to the reference and the analysis. If a large share of that, approximately $60 billion, is in hospitals, it could raise hospital charges by 20% overall.[11] Then there is the assumed amount used by underinsured citizens, which is $126 billion. What percentage does the underinsured patient pay, and what percentage are other patients or, in fact, every employed or retired American paying?

The funding for a universal healthcare program in the United States can be simplified by extending an improved Medicare as a National Health Program to the entire population while also eliminating high co-payments and deductibles and providing universal drug coverage. This National Health Program would be a publicly financed, publicly accountable, and locally controlled healthcare program which would deliver the best care for every American with the lowest administrative costs and overhead. This program would allow patients freedom of choice, doctors the freedom to treat, and hospitals the freedom to care for all people. As I have pointed out, providing healthcare to every American will be the real means to release competitive forces on quality and service to patients.

A cap on total administrative costs should be placed at less than 10% of total health spending. Currently, Medicare has about 2% administrative costs, but the government can place additional administrative costs onto the physicians, hospitals, nursing homes and others. This costly and unnecessary excess administration in the U.S. must be significantly reduced. Placing a cap on the total administrative costs (providers, payers, and patients) will redirect more money to the actual care of the patients. Patients need and providers can deliver more access to medical services if bureaucracy was significantly reduced.

Medical and dental school educational costs need to be covered for students who wish to enter the professions. I am not asking for more money for physicians or dentists, but I am asking for the elimination of large provider debts which must be paid with after-tax dollars and are then passed on to the patients and the insurance industry for years to come.

There surely will be a protest to any thought of new taxes for an expanded Medicare or National Health Program. There is every reason to believe, however, that in a competently designed and executed program, the new taxes will be less than the premiums and out-of-pocket costs all Americans now pay. Businesses currently encumbered with expensive employer-based health costs will realize significant savings under this proposal leading to higher wages for employees or larger profits for owner-investors. Those businesses that currently fail to provide employer-based health insurance would soon realize healthier and more productive workers. Self-employed Americans, like George the carpenter and Sam the farmer, will finally have decent and reliable coverage.

The federal government could become the single-payer by including current taxes paid into the Medicare program and other government health-care funding sources plus implementing a new National Health Program. Presently Medicare is funded by a 1.45% tax on employers and employees. In 1998, this generated $213 billion while Medicare spent $216.6 billion or 19% of total U.S. health spending. Out-of-pocket costs were $199.5 billion or 17% of the total. Reducing out-of-pocket costs to a maximum of 10% of total income for every individual and family would lower out-of-pocket costs to $99.75 billion. In 1998, all levels of government, including Medicare and health insurance for government employees, paid $585 billion or 51% of the total with tax dollars. To generate the same amount of total spending, $1,149.1 billion using 1998 to model the National Health Program (NHP), an increased tax of $448.9 billion would be required. This would supplant insurance premiums of $375 billion, out-of-pocket costs of 99.5 billion and other private funding of 38.8 billion. The new tax would be $57.5 billion less than the former payments. See Figure Twenty-six on the following page.

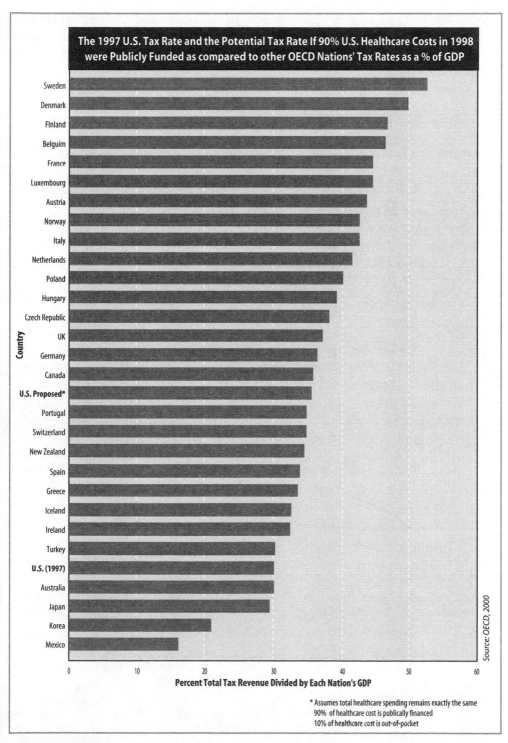

The 1997 U.S. Tax Rate and the Potential Tax Rate If 90% U.S. Healthcare Costs in 1998 were Publicly Funded as compared to other OECD Nations' Tax Rates as a % of GDP

Percent Total Tax Revenue Divided by Each Nation's GDP

Source: OECD, 2000

* Assumes total healthcare spending remains exactly the same
90% of healthcare cost is publically financed
10% of healthcare cost is out-of-pocket

Figure Twenty-six

The dynamics of the savings versus the new taxes are represented in the following table, using 1998 to model the initial year of enactment. The information is from the OECD Health 2000 Database; from the Bureau of the Census, and from HCFA. The basic assumptions to the extension of the 1998 model are:

1. The program recommended is strongly initiated and realizes the estimated savings.

2. Healthcare inflation is reduced to 1.86 %; economic growth is 3%; total growth in healthcare spending, including new use, is 3%.

3. Up to one and a half million persons employed in the industry's bureaucracy are displaced and are converted to healthcare occupations. The retraining cost averages $20,000 per person, assuming community college involvement.

4. The present Medicare and new NHP tax total is 9% of personal income, split between employers and employees. The other tax support remains in place.

5. Nurses are accorded an increase in salary over the inflation rate of 15% over three years beginning in the second year.

6. The buyout of for-profit healthcare businesses is estimated to be $88 billion. Straight line amortization is $12.57 billion for seven years. The interest is 6% per year, assumed to be at the long-term bond rate.

7. Public health, VA, military, and research continue to be funded through their present channels and operate separately. The VA system could be integrated in the future.

8. The capital items of construction and a buy-out of for-profit institutions are separated from the current expenses in the 1998 model. As many financial commentators and others have noted, government accounting is remiss in often combining the two. The current part of construction is the amortization loans for the purchase of assets. This is assumed to be included in the revenue of hospitals and where applicable for doctors' groups and other institutions. The capital expenses for facilities construction are therefore deducted from the 1998 model, and the buy-out expenses are not included in current expenditures, so as not to distort analyses.[12]

Analysis of Taxes and Savings in a National Healthcare Program

	1998	1999	2000	2001	2002
1998 expenditure	-$1,149.10	-$1,183.57	-$1,219.08	-$1,255.65	-$1,293.32
Less capital included	15.5	15.79	16.08	16.38	16.69
New rights	-110.2	-113.51	-116.91	-120.42	-124.03
Retraining	-20	-10	—	—	—
Tuition	-2	-2	-2	-2	-2
Nurses increase	—	-4.3	-4.3	-4.3	—
Sub total	**-$1,265.80**	**-$1,297.59**	**-$1,326.21**	**-$1,365.99**	**-$1,402.67**
NHP SAVINGS:					
Reduced Rx Marketing	10.9	10.9	10.9	10.9	10.9
Insurance	43.9	43.9	43.9	43.9	43.9
Defensive medicine	22.9	22.9	22.9	22.9	22.9
Excess admininstration	46.5	46.5	46.5	46.5	46.5
Reduced Illnesses	16	40	64	88	112
Sub Total	**140.2**	**164.2**	**188.2**	**212.2**	**236.2**
NHP NET COST:	-1,125.60	-1,133.39	-1,138.01	-1,153.79	-1,166.47
NHP PAYMENTS:					
Lower out-of-pocket	99.75	102.74	105.82	109.00	112.27
Present tax support	369.2	380.28	391.68	403.43	415.54
Present Medicare	216.6	223.10	229.79	236.68	243.79
Other private	1.6	1.63	1.66	1.69	1.72
Sub Total	**685.55**	**706.12**	**727.30**	**749.12**	**771.59**
New funds needed	-$440.05	-$427.27	-$410.71	-$404.67	-$394.87
NHP TAX 6.1%	448.9	462.37	476.24	490.53	505.24
Program net	8.85	35.09	65.53	85.85	110.37
Program balance	8.85	43.94	109.47	195.33	305.69
GDP	8277.9	8526.2	8782.0	9045.5	9316.8
% GDP	13.60%	13.29%	12.96%	12.76%	12.52%
Capital Accounts:					
New facilities	15.5	15.79	16.08	16.38	16.69
Buyout interest	—	6.10	4.50	3.70	3.10
Buyout amort.	—	12.5	12.5	12.5	12.5

This analysis leaves existing taxes in place and institutes a 6.1% National Health Program tax, raising the total Medicare tax to 9%. There is an alternative, namely a complete restructuring of healthcare taxes and implementing a direct tax for the entire public funding of the National Health Program. This would reflect a gigantic restructuring and would reduce current income and real estate taxes. The "sin" taxes on tobacco and alcohol would be continued, but medical treatments to all patients addicted to or suffering from tobacco or alcohol-related illness would be available.

I favor one well-planned, but tumultuous year in which the whole conversion happens, and this should occur as soon as possible. The uninsured and underinsured get their full-scale quality healthcare. The for-profit insurance companies bow and leave. The not-for-profit staff model HMOs reestablish themselves. The health employees or insurance personnel displaced through this program enactment choose their retraining. They quickly enter into health service areas, where they are already needed. Real estate taxes and others fall; the new healthcare tax is inaugurated. The new system begins paying, with banks financing the transition under government guarantees. Hard to do? Yes. But, this will save the most lives and the most money in the most expeditious manner. The use of the present tax-funding sources and structure simplifies this policy change and allows for future adjustments.

The healthcare lobby will use its established ability to manipulate public opinion and its political power to claim that this new policy would be "socialized medicine," add waiting lines, increase rationing, stifle new technology, set price controls, limit competition, worsen quality, increase taxes, raise costs because it's "free," continue inequality, reduce individual responsibility, and be "un-American."

I have tried to answer many of these criticisms throughout the chapters of this book. The proposed National Healthcare Program is not "socialized medicine." Patients would have the freedom to choose their physician, specialists and other providers, their hospital and their pharmacy. Competition of quality and service will flourish under universal health insurance. Physicians, dentists, and other providers would have the freedom to practice their specialty, choose their practice location, and their practice setting (fee-for-service, salaried or employed, solo, group practice, clinic or hospital). When there is full access to the doctor or institution of choice, then the doctors and the institutions have to compete by providing quality service and treatment, far from the present market-driven or money-oriented system. It is a longer-term competition of service and quality, which is meaningful in healthcare. To an allegation of universal care causing waiting lines I have a response. People in this country die sooner relative to the comparison nations, the ultimate waiting line. And, nearly 70% of the uninsured adult patients in poor health fail to see a doctor in one year. I would definitely call that an impressive waiting line.

A National Health Program will not stifle medical technology. The U.S. defense industry is federally funded for national defense, and America has the most high-tech military in the world. The defense industry manufacturers are private companies making reasonable profits. Japan has had national health insurance for almost forty years and also has more MRI and CAT scanners per million population than does the U.S. They probably also develop more new medications per unit of population.[13]

And medical care is not "free" in the United States. We have the third highest out-of-pocket costs in the world and with current market-driven forces these numbers will only climb further. Nearly every insurance company or government official seems to call for passing more of the health costs onto the patients. Only 54% of private-sector workers were offered coverage from their own employer in 1998, down from 65% one decade earlier. And approximately only a third of large employers are offering their retirees any health benefits, down from nearly 50% one decade earlier.[14] I hear and see daily from patients complaining about their higher deductibles, co-pays, and insurance premiums or the lack of coverage. Medical care in the United States is anything but free to these people. But the reality or fear of high medical costs can truly harm patients, for this book is loaded with real human stories and tragedies that could have been prevented with universal "free" care.

I also commonly hear some leaders criticize a national health program by claiming one-size-does-not-fit-all in healthcare. I disagree when it comes to a national health system. Doctors, nurses and other health providers should treat every individual patient according to his clinical condition and medical problems and not according to the patient's type of insurance or wallet size. In a court of law the medical profession is expected to meet the "standard of care" for each and every patient. Do insured or rich patients have a different standard of care when compared to the uninsured or not-so-rich patients? And what would happen if all government officials, doctors, hospital and pharmaceutical company executives, the wealthy and their families had the same coverage and access to medical care as all other Americans? I believe these political, medical and economic leaders would make sure the system works and meets their individual and family's needs and all others too.

Prices will be controlled by the national program. Healthcare is treated as a regulated monopoly in the other democratic OECD nations. A nation's health system is a fundamental social service, as is the provision of clean water, electric power, public education, police and fire protection, too important to be left to pure market whims. The differences between the other nations' health systems are similar to national policies regarding electricity. Some nations have publicly owned utilities akin to government hospitals with all doctors on salary. In others, the electric power generation is local or private in a regulated monopoly. That is like hospitals being owned by local communities, with doctors in their own practices. Only in the United States would a monopoly be deregulated to produce the present energy crisis in California.

Healthcare subtly has all of the characteristics of a monopoly, and the lobby is trying to hang onto its yet to be regulated status. As in dealing with a monopoly, prices are not forced on the companies participating. Rather, a negotiation to allow full returns on investment with incentives to expand capabilities must result. In the final analysis, a healthier and more economically sound health system will benefit all individuals of a democratic society.

The current system in America cannot save patients from profit-driven and money-oriented healthcare. A truly universal National Healthcare Program, granting the right to decent healthcare for all people in this nation, can place the patients first and overcome the market-driven and incremental reform policies. I call on all Americans to end this national embarrassment. The United States must take the leap and join the rest of the democratic countries of the world in affirming the right to decent healthcare for all of its citizens and granting universal healthcare regardless of race, sex, color, age, origin, disability, orientation or ability to pay, both in and outside the hospital. There is much work to be done in this endeavor.

An elected official in our community once was quoted in the local paper as saying, "Health is a person's responsibility. If you don't care about it, why should I care about it?"[15]

In response, I offer Deuteronomy 15:7-11, *If there is among you anyone in need, a member of your community in any of your towns within the land ...do not be hard-hearted or tight-fisted toward your needy neighbor. You should rather open your hand, willingly lending enough to meet the need, whatever it may be.*

Has the heart and soul of America been hardened to the point it cannot provide decent healthcare to all people living within the land? I surely hope this is not the case, but it surely seems to be the effect. Even "healthy individuals" will have unforeseen, accidental, or unexplained illnesses and require help. As for the rest of us, who may sometimes make poor choices or poor health decisions, we too will need medical care. All of society eventually pays heavily when healthcare is denied, both directly and indirectly, as I have tried to demonstrate. Health is much more than an individual's responsibility. The issue of healthcare in the United States is a matter of social consciousness.

As Quentin Young M.D. has rightly stated, "The present system is awash in tragedy. It has to be righted. Everybody in. Nobody out."

THE AFTERWORD

A voice of one calling:"In the desert prepare the way of the Lord; make straight in the wilderness..."

Isaiah 40:3-5. The New International Version

While I sometimes feel like a lone voice calling out in the desert wilderness of the American health scene, I know that there are many others calling out also. Many physicians, nurses, clergy, educators, economists, politicians, patients and others are trying to change our broken and sick healthcare system. Healthcare is a human right, and this nation cannot lead the democratic world until this basic human right is granted to every human being living in this nation. I find our market-driven system unjust and inhumane to the very people it supposedly serves, the patients.

I know many Americans feel they cannot change a system or make a difference, but I strongly object. It will take much effort, courage and faith to repair a wrong. We remember that the Declaration of Independence was imperfect in the beginning. Many of the original authors of this great document had slaves of their own, and all of the writers failed to mention women and children when they stated, "All men are created equal."

This nation has had to rise up when liberty and justice for all people has been subverted or withheld. Many people have risked their lives and faced extreme hardship over their beliefs in truth and justice. The Civil War nearly broke this country apart over slavery and the right to own human beings. Decades later women marched the streets for the simple right to vote. And many decades after that minorities had to protest peacefully and sometimes even violently to bring true Civil Rights to all people. The end of the Vietnam War only came after thousands of students, mothers and many others suffered much pain and loss. Some even lost their lives to bullets flying at Kent State. What will patients have to do to obtain the right to quality, affordable, accessible healthcare for all people in this great nation? How many community hospitals will be closed? I hope the American people will not see more violence, murders and human suffering. Too many Americans are already paying a heavy price of premature illness, disability and death from a failing and sick health system.

Let us make this the enormous human rights issue the issue of the new millennium in the United States and resurrect the patients from the money-oriented and market-driven healthcare system. Talk to your neighbors, elected officials and healthcare workers, including your doctor. Browse the many websites such as www.pnhp.org, www.nofreelunch.org, www.healthcare-forall.org, www.everybodyinnobodyout.org, www.amsa.org, and follow the links. The truth must come forward for the patients and society. I urge you to write to your local, state and national legislators calling for implementation of a local, state or national health program, which covers all people.

Currently, federal legislation before the Congress includes H.R.1200, the American Health Security Act of 2001, sponsored by Representative Jim McDermott. The Act calls for the provision of healthcare for every American, to control costs and enhance the quality of the healthcare system. The other is H.CON.RES.99, sponsored by Representative John Conyers, Jr., directing Congress to enact legislation by October 2004 that provides access to comprehensive healthcare for all Americans. And finally an important proposal was made by Massachusetts Representative John Tierney to fund the research and development of state healthcare plans. The bill titled States' Right to Innovate in Healthcare Act, would allow states to experiment with a universal system.

Current legislation in New York includes universal single-payer bills S 3575 and A 5712 that have been proposed yearly since 1997. Sponsored by Assemblyman Colton and Senator Stavisky. No action was taken by the Senate Committee on Health nor by the Assembly Committee on Insurance by the end of the 2000 sessions. What are our New York elected officials waiting for? The bills would "authorize and direct the commissioners of the State Insurance Fund to establish a single-payer healthcare plan." Another plan proposed February 18, 2000, is S 6653, New York Health Plan that would provide universal health coverage, access to and choice of healthcare providers for all residents of New York, controls on healthcare costs, development of healthcare services and public financing. The plan calls for a board of governors to administer the plan, with partial funding from premiums placed on employers.

Many other states may have similar legislation awaiting action by their elected officials. In the State of Maine, the House passed bill, LD 1277, an Act to establish a single-payer Healthcare System, on May 21, 2001, by a margin of 80-58. The bill would guarantee comprehensive healthcare coverage for every Maine resident through a public financing system. "Maine has taken the lead in healthcare in this country with the first-in-the-nation prescription drug law to rein in the pharmaceutical industry. Now our national leadership on this issue is bringing universal healthcare to the brink of passage. As Maine goes, so goes the nation," further remarked State Representative Paul Volenik. One bold state will finally take a leap of faith and implement a truly universal healthcare program. I believe they will succeed in their mission, and many other states will soon follow.

If American families want to continue spending at least 40% more for healthcare compared to the rest of the industrialized world while obtaining only mediocre results, then don't change a thing. Keep the incrementalism movement going; it only channels more money to those in the healthcare industry, of which many are for-profit. But if you truly want the best healthcare for all people, including yourself and your family, then support a multpayer universal system similar to the French or the Japanese. And, if Americans wish to stop wasting the nearly $100 billion a year on multiple insurance payers and the administrative absurdities, then support a single-payer National Healthcare Program. And lastly, I appeal to every American, do not turn your head and look away from the millions of Americans who are suffering unnecessary illness, premature disability, and early death from our sick health system. For that truly would continue to be "As Sick As It Gets."

THE REFERENCES

The key abbreviations are:

AMNews: *American Medical News*
BMJ: *British Medical Journal*
HCFA: Health Care Financing Administration
JAMA: *Journal of the American Medical Association*
MMWR: *Morbidity and Mortality Weekly Report*
MSSNYU: Medical Society of the State of NY
NEJM: *New England Journal of Medicine*
SAUS 2000: *Statistical Abstract of the United States, 2000*

The full OECD Health Data 2000 reference is:

Organization for Economic Cooperation and Development
Health Policy Unit
2 rue Andre Pascal
F-75775 Paris Cedex 16
Fax: (33) 1 44 30 63 61 E-mail: sante.contact@oecd.org

INTRODUCTION

1. Stapleton, Stephanie. "Where's the Nurse?" *AMNews* (June 18, 2001): 50.
2. Forster, Jeff. "Reality Check: Which Doctors are Heading For the Exits." *Medical Economics*, (August 21, 2000) and "And Then There Were None; The Coming Physician Supply Problem." California Med. Assoc. (July 2001).
3. CBS News Poll, (July 13–14, 2001): <www.pollingreport.com/health>.
4. WHO, Center for Health Economics Research, 18 (1993): 6.
5. Organization for Economic Cooperation and Development, Health Data 2000, and HCFA *Healthcare Financing Review*, (Winter 1999): SAUS 2000 tables 151/2.
6. OECD, Health Data 2000.
7. WHO, World Health Organization Report 2000. <www.who.int>.
8. Aston, G. "Number of Uninsured Down, But Struggle Continues." *AMNews*, (October 16, 2000).
9. OECD, Health Data 2000.
10. <www.statehealthfacts.kff.org>. (June 1, 2001)
11. National Center for Health Statistics, "New Study of Patterns of Death in U.S.," (February 23, 1998).

CHAPTER 1

1. Aston, G. "Number of Uninsured Down, But Struggle Continues." *AMNews*, (October 16, 2000).
2. Kaiser Commission Report, "Uninsured in America." (May 2000).
3. U.S. Census Bureau Health Insurance Data.
4. American College of Physicians/American Society of Internal Medicine (ACP/ASIM). (8/31/01): <www.acponline.org/uninsured/index.html>.
5. Ayanian, John Z. MD, MPP. Weissman, Joel S. PhD. Schneider, Eric C. MD, MSc. Ginsburg, Jack

A. MPE. Zaslavsky, Alan M. PhD "Unmet Health Needs of Uninsured Adults in the United States." JAMA, 284 (16) (October 25, 2000): 2061–9.

6. JAMA, 265 (1991): 374.

7. American College of Physicians/ American Society of Internal Medicine (ACP/ASIM). (8/31/01): <www.acponline.org/uninsured/index.html>.

8. Kessler, Ronald; Davis, Roger; Foster, David F. MD. Van Rompay, Maria; Walters, Ellen; Wilkey, Sonja; Kaptchuk, Ted; Eisenberg, David. "Long-Term Trends in the Use of Complementary and Alternative Medical Therapies in the United States." *Annals Int Med* 135(4)(2001): 262–8.

9. Steinhauer, Jennifer, *The New York Times*, (October 25, 2000).

10. <www.statehealthfacts.kff.org>. (June 1, 2001).

11. International Labor Organization, (1999).

12. Ayanian, John Z. MD, MPP. Weissman, Joel S. PhD. Schneider, Eric C. MD, MSc. Ginsburg, Jack A. MPE. Zaslavsky, Alan M. PhD "Unmet Health Needs of Uninsured Adults in the United States." JAMA, 284 (16) (October 25, 2000): 2061–9.

13. Garrett, Bowen; Holahan, John. "Health Insurance Coverage After Welfare." *Health Affairs*, 19 (1) (2000): 175.

14. <www.statehealthfacts.kff.org>. (6/1/01).

15. Ayanian, John Z. MD, MPP. Weissman, Joel S. PhD. Schneider, Eric C. MD, MSc. Ginsburg, Jack A. MPE. Zaslavsky, Alan M. PhD "Unmet Health Needs of Uninsured Adults in the United States." JAMA, 284 (16) (October 25, 2000): 2061–9.

16. Health for All of Western New York, Inc., "Health Risk Assessment Survey," (1999).

17. Lyons, Albert S. MD. *Medicine, An Illustrated History*, Harry Abrams, Inc. New York. (1978): 360.

CHAPTER 2

1. In 1993 the National Health Interview Survey (NHIS) asked questions about unmet medical needs in the population age range of 18 to 64 inclusive. The responses were distributed in various ways including those who had no insurance and those who had private, public or "other" insurance. Based on population as reported in SAUS 1995 table 16 (for 1994) and the total of uninsured persons in Table 169 the total of uninsured persons was 29.8 million in the age group or18.7%. There were 114.9 million with private insurance and 15.8 million with Medicare disability or Medicaid. Of the uninsured 41.7 % reported an unmet medical need, but so also did 14.4% of the privately insured, 32% of the government insured. This bears witness to the OECD Health Data 2000 report that in fact 55% of Americans are not fully insured. In the age group the total uninsured with unmet needs was 12,426,600. The total of insured who had unmet needs was 21,601,600. These were 7.8% and 13.6% of the total of the age group respectively. To estimate the number of seriously underinsured the percent of those who needed immediate care but could not get it was used. The projections from the sample were that 3,129,000 uninsured persons could not get such care and 3,545, 000 with insurance were in the same circumstance at one time during the year. There are no clear data for the young people and children under 18. In this age group, 9.6 million had no insurance and 16.6 million were on Medicaid. And well over 10 million Medicare patients over the age of 64 lack any prescription coverage. Thus the estimate that the total of uninsured and seriously underinsured Americans is nearly the same or 43 million uninsured and 42 million underinsured.

2. National Center for Health Statistics on Oral Health, (2000) and Iglehart, John K., "Medicare and Prescription Drugs." *NEJM* 344 (13) (March 29, 2001): 1010–1015.

3. Aston, G. "Number of Uninsured Down, But Struggle Continues." *AMNews*, (October 16, 2000).

4. OECD, Health Data 2000.

5. American Association of Retired Persons (AARP), (March 1998).

6. Hay Group Survey of Medium Labor Firms, (April 1999).

7. Wrich, J., Audit findings submitted to CBO, (March 1998).
8. "Historical statistics and statistical abstract of the U.S. Bureau Justice Statistics." *The New York Times*, (October 23, 1998).
9. *Harrison's Principles of Internal Medicine*, McGraw-Hill, Inc. 13 (1994): 142, 2270–1.
10. Norton's Bankruptcy Advisor, (May 2000).
11. Freund, Deborah; Willison, Don; Reeher, Grant; Cosby, Jarold; Ferraro, Amy; O'Brien, Bernie. "Outpatient Pharmaceuticals and the Elderly: Policies in Seven Nations." *Health Affairs*, 19 (3) (2000): 259–66.
12. *Consumer Reports*, (September 2000).
13. Himmelstein, David; Woolhandler, Steffie; Hellander, Ida. *Bleeding the Patient: The Consequences of Corporate Healthcare*. Common Courage Press, Monroe Maine. (2001): 216–7.
14. *Annals of Long-term Care*, (Nov/Dec 2000): 18.

CHAPTER 3

1. Rector, Thomas S. PhD. "Exhaustion of Drug Benefits and Disenrollment of Medicare Beneficiaries From Managed Care Organizations." *JAMA*, 283 (16) (2000): 2163–7.
2. Gawande, Atul A.;. Blendon, Robert J; Brodie, Mollyann; Benson, John M.; Levitt, Larry; Hugick, Larry. "Does Dissatisfaction With Health Plans Stem From Having No Choices?" *Health Affairs*, 17 (5) (1998): 184.
3. Cunningham, Peter; Kohn, Linda. "Health Plan Switching: Choice or Circumstance?" *Health Affairs*, 19 (3) (2000): 158.
4. Commonwealth Fund Survey, (1998): <www.cmwf.org/index.asp>.
5. *AMNews* (June 25, 2001): 5–6.
6. American College of Physicians/ American Society of Internal Medicine (ACP/ASIM). (8/31/01): <www.acponline.org/uninsured/index.html>.
7. <www.statehealthfacts.kff.org>.

CHAPTER 4

1. Hamburger/McGinley, *The Wall Street Journal*, (November 9, 2000), consumer reports (September 2000) and Kuttner, Robert. "Toward Universal Coverage." *The Washington Post*, National Weekly Edition, (July 20–27, 1998).
2. <www.phrma.org>, (3/15/01).
3. DeAngelis, Catherine D. MD, MPH. "Conflict of Interest and the Public Trust."
    JAMA, 284 (17) (November 1, 2000): 2237–8.
4. <www.phrma.org>, (3/15/01).
5. Ibid.
6. *Consumer Reports*, (October 1993): 673.
7. AMA, *Council of Ethical and Judicial Affairs*, Edition 1996–1977: 118, AMNews 44 (25) (2001): 19 and <www.ama-assn.org/go/ethicalgifts>, (9/14/01).
8. Steinman, Michael A., MD, "Gifts to Physicians in the Consumer Marketing Era." *JAMA*, 284 (November 1, 2000): 2243.
9. Wazana, Ashley, MD, "Physicians and the Pharmaceutical Industry: Is a Gift Ever Just a Gift?" *JAMA*, 282 (January 19,2000): 373–80.
10. <www.nofreelunch.org>, (4/1/01).

11. Ziegler, Michael; Lew, Pauline; Singer, Brian. "The Accuracy of Drug Information from Pharmaceutical Sales Representatives." *JAMA*, 273 (1995): 1296–8.

12. Adams, Christopher, "Doctors on the Run." *The Wall Street Journal*.

13. Iglehart, John K. "Medicare and Prescription Drugs." *NEJM*, 344 (13) (2001): 1010–5.

14. *Journal of Family Practice*, 45 (1997): 494–9.

15. Bell, Robert A., Ph.D.; Wilkes, Michael S., MD, Ph.D.; Kravitz, Richard L., MD, MSPH, "Advertisement-Induced Prescription Drug Requests: Patients' Anticipated Reaction to a Physician Who Refuses." *Journal of Family Practice*, 48 (1999): 446–452.

16. *The New York Times*, "How to Lower the Cost of Drugs." (January 3, 2001).

17. *Worst Pills/Best Pills*, 7 (6) (2001): 47.

18. *Fortune 500*, "Ranking for 1999."

19. Congressional Research Service, CBO, (December 13,1999).

20. Pear, Robert, "Rise in Health Care Cost Rests Largely on Drug Price." *The New York Times*, (November 14, 2000).

21. Pear, Robert, " Rise in Health Care Cost Rests Largely on Drug Price." *The New York Times*, (November 14, 2000).

22. Moynihan, Ray; Bero, Lisa; Ross-Degnan, Dennis; Henry, David; Lee, Kirby; Watkins, Judy; May, Connie; Soumerai, Stephen B., "Coverage by the New Media of the Benefits and Risks of Medications." *NEJM*, 324 (22) (June 1, 2000): 1645–50.

23. Boyd, Elizabeth A., Ph.D.; Bero, Lisa A., Ph.D., "Assessing Faculty Financial Relationships with Industry: A Case Study." *JAMA*, 248 (November 1, 2000): 2209–14.

24. Albert, Michelle; Danielson, Ellie; Rifai, Nader; Ridker, Paul. "Effect of Statin Therapy on C-Reactive Protein Levels." *JAMA*, 286 (1) (2001): 64–70.

25. Foubister, V. "Getting Prescriptions to the People." *AMNews*, (Oct 23/30, 2000): 11.

26. AARP, <www.aarp.org/egi-bin//myaarp/articledetail>, (2/4/01).

27. Poisal, John A.; Murray, Lauren, "Growing Differences Between Medicare Beneficiaries With and Without Drug Coverage." *Health Affairs*, 20 (2) (2001): 74–85.

28. Long, S.H., "Universal Health Insurance and Uninsured People: Effects on Use and Cost: Report to Congress." Washington, DC., Office of Technology Assessment and Congressional Research Survey, Library of Congress. (August 5, 1994).

29. ACP/ASIM. <www.acponline.org/uninsured/index.html>.

CHAPTER 5

1. Levit, K et al. Health Spending in 1998: Signals of Change." *Health Affairs*, 19 (1) (2000); 124–32 and Fox, D; Fronstin, P. "Public Spending for Health Care Approaches 60 Percent." *Health Affairs*, 19 (2) (2000): 271–3 and Himmelstein, David; Woolhandler, Steffie; Hellander, Ida. *Bleeding the Patient: The Consequences of Corporate Healthcare*. Common Courage Press, Monroe Maine. (2001): 159. Depending on which reference quoted, public funding in 1998 can range from a low of 45% (Levit) to a high of 64.1% (Himmelstein). 56% was estimated by Fox using the Levit study and including the public's portion of public employees' private health insurance premiums ($63.1 billion) and tax expenditures, defined as tax collections forgone as a result of health and social policy carried out through tax law ($124.8 billion). At a minimum I believe any estimate must include the governmentt's portion of public employees' private health insurance bringing the total to 51%.

2. *AMNews*, "U.S. Census Bureau Health Insurance Data." (October 16, 2000).

3. Commerce Department. <www.census.gov/press-release/www.1999/CB99-178.html>, (February 21, 2000).

4. *MSSNY News of New York*, (December 2000): 8.

5. "And Then There Were None; The Coming Physician Supply Problem." *California Med. Assoc.*, (July 2001).

CHAPTER 6

1. Lovern, Ed. *Modern Healthcare Magazine*, (January 8, 2001).

2. *AMNews*, (November 20, 2000).

3. Himmelstein, David; Woolhandler, Steffie; Hellander, Ida. *Bleeding the Patient: The Consequences of Corporate Healthcare*, Common Courage Press, Monroe Maine. (2001): 195–6.

4. Ibid.

5. *Time Magazine*, (April 28, 2001): 41.

6. Naradzay, Jerome F., MD., "Into the Deep Well: The Evolution of Medical School Loan Debt." JAMA, 280 (21) (1998): 1881–3.

7. Stockewell, A., *The Guerilla Guide to Mastering Student Loan Debt*, Harper Perennial, NY, NY, (1997).

8. Himmelstein, David; Woolhandler, Steffie; Hellander, Ida. *Bleeding the Patient: The Consequences of Corporate Healthcare*, Common Courage Press, Monroe Maine. (2001): 48.

9. Baransky, Barbara Ph.D.,: Jonas, Harry S., MD.; Etzel, Sylvia I., "Educational Programs in U.S. Medical School, 1999–2000." JAMA, 248 (9) (2000): 1114–9 and Krakower, J; Coble, T; Williams, D; Jones, R. "Review of United States Medical School Finances, 1998–1999." JAMA, 248 (9) (2000): 1127–9.

10. *AMNews*, 44(9) (2001).

11. Studdert, David; Brennan, Troyen. "No-Fault Compensation for Medical Injuries: The Prospect for Error Prevention." JAMA, 286 (2) (2001): 217–228.

12. Brett, Allan S., "New Guidelines for Coding Physicians' Services—A Step Backward." NEJM, 339 (23) (1998): 1705–8.

13. Doescher, M.; Franks, P.: Banthin, J.; Clancy, C. "Supplemental Insurance and Mortality in Elderly Americans." *Archives of Family Medicine*, 9 (2000): 251–7.

14. *Journal of the American Women's Medical Association*, 55 (1) (2000): 37–38.

15. Starfield, Barbara MD, MPH, "Is U.S. Health Really the Best in the World?" JAMA 284 (4) (2000): 483–5.

16. Larkin, Howard, *AMNews*, (December 27, 1999).

17. Nelson, Alan R. MD "Medicine: Business or profession, art or science?" *American Journal of Obstetrics and Gynecology*, 178 (1998): 755–8.

18. U.S. Census 2000.

19. Freeman, HP, "Racial Injustice in Healthcare." NEJM, 342 (14) (April 6, 2000): 1045–1047.

20. Simon, Steven R.; Pan, Richard, JD; Sullivan, Amy M.; Clark-Chiarelli, Nancy; Connelly, Maureen T.; Peters, Antoinette S.; Singer, Judith D.; Inui, Thomas S.; Block, Susan D., "View of Managed Care—A Survey of Students, Residents, Faculty and Deans at Medical Schools in the United States." NEJM, 342 (12) (1999): 928–36.

21. Studdert, David M. LLB, ScD, MPH; Brennan, Troyen A., MD, JD, MPH, "No-Fault Compensation for Medical Injuries: The Prospect for Error Prevention." JAMA, 286 (2) (2001): 217–228.

22. Emanuel, Ezekiel J. MD, Ph.D.; Fairclough, Diane L. DPH; Slustman, Julia BA; Emanuel, Linda L. MD, Ph.D., "Understanding Economic and Other Burdens of Terminal Illness: The Experience of Patients and Their Caregivers." *Annals of Internal Medicine*, 132 (2000): 451–9.

23. Williams, Walter E., *Ideas of Liberty*, (October 2000): 63–4.

24. Nelson, Alan R. MD "Medicine: Business or profession, art or science?" *American Journal of Obstetrics and Gynecology*, 178 (1998): 755–8.

Chapter 7

1. OECD, Health Data 2000.
2. Ibid.
3. Roemer, M.I., *National Health Systems of the World*, Oxford University Press New York: (1991).
4. Lazar, Harold; Fitzgerald, Carmel; Ahmad, Tazeen; Bao, Yusheng; Colton, Theodore; Shapira, Oz ; Shemin, Richard. "Early discharge after coronary artery bypass graft surgery: Are patients really going home earlier?" *Jr Thoracic Card Surg*, 121 (5) (2001): 943–50.
5. *Oxford Review*, "Economic Policy." 5 (1) (1989): 89.
6. Shi, L.; Starfield, B.; Kennedy, B.; Kawachi, I. "Income Inequality, Primary Care, and Health Indicators." *Journal of Family Practice*, 48 (4) (April 1999): 275–84.
7. Wilkinson, R.G., "Income distribution and life expectancy," *BMJ* 304 (1992): 165–8 and Kaplan, G.; Pamuk, E.; Lynch, J.; Cohen, R.; Balfour, J. "Inequality in Income and Mortality in the United States: Analysis of Mortality and Potential Pathways." BMJ, 312 (7037) (1996): 995–1003.
8. *NEJM*, 329 (1993): 103–109.
9. OECD, Health Data 2000.
10. Quinn, Michell, *The Orange County Register*, (April 10, 2001).
11. Shi, L.; Starfield, B.; Kennedy, B.; Kawachi, I. "Income Inequality, Primary Care, and Health Indicators." *Journal of Family Practice*, 48 (4) (April 1999): 275–84.
12. WHO Report 2000.
13. Ibid.
14. Speed, Sir Keith, Personal communication. (July 19, 2001).
15. OECD, Health Data 2000.
16. Himmelstein, David; Woolhandler, Steffie; Hellander, Ida. *Bleeding the Patient: The Consequences of Corporate Healthcare*. Common Courage Press, Monroe Maine. (2001): 203.
17. WHO Report 2000, Annex Table 8.
18. Blendon, Robert; Schoen, Cathy; Donelan, Karen; Osborn, Robin; DesRoches, Catherine; Scoles, Kimberly; Davis, Karen; Binns, Katherine; Zapert, Kinga. "Physicians' Views On Quality Of Care: A Five-Country Comparison." *Health Affairs*, 2001; 20(3): 233–41.
19. Southham Medical Database. Canadian Institute for Health Information, 2000. <www.cihi.ca>.
20. *AMNews* (April 9, 2001): 18., *AMNews*, (April 16, 2001): 11–4.
21. Canadian Medical Association. Masterfile 2000./AMA Data Resources Physicians Statistics: Now. <www.amassn.org/ama/pub/category/2688.html>.
22. Forster, Jeff. "Reality Check: Which Doctors are Heading For the Exits." *Medical Economics*, (August 21, 2000).
23. "And Then There Were None; The Coming Physician Supply Problem." *California Med. Assoc.*, (July 2001).
24. Iglehart, John K., "Revisiting the Canadian Health Care System." *NJEM*, 342 (26) (June 29, 2000): 2007–12.
25. OECH, Health Data 2000.
26. Rosenthal, Thomas C. MD. Fox, Chester MD. "Access to Health Care for the Rural Elderly." *JAMA*, 284 (16) (2000): 2034–6.
27. Ibid.
28. Canadian Medical Association. Masterfile 2000./AMA Data Resources Physicians Statistics: Now. <http://www.amassn.org/ama/pub/category/2688.html>.
29. *Medical Economics*, (August 2000) and Kraker, Daniel, Research Associate, Institute for Local Self-Reliance.

30. OECD, Health Data 2000.

31. Fielding, Jonathan E., "Lessons from France—Vive la Difference: The French Healthcare System and U.S. Health System Reform." *JAMA,* 270 (6) 11 (Aug. 1993): 748–756.

32. Ibid.

33. CBS News Poll (July 13–14, 1999).

34. Annas, George. "Human Rights and Health—The Universal Declaration of Human Rights at 50." *NEJM,* 339 (24) (1998): 1778–82.

35. WHO Report 2000, Annex Table 8.

36. Tamblyn, R; Laprise, R; Hanley, J; Abrahamowicz, M; Scott, S; Mayo, N; Hurley, J; Grad, R; Latimer, E; Perreault, R; McLeod, P; Huang, A; Larochelle, P; Mallet, L. "Adverse Events Associated With Prescription Drug Cost-Sharing Among Poor and Elderly Persons." *JAMA,* 285 (4) (1/24–31/01): 421–9.

37. Doescher, M.; Franks, P.: Banthin, J.; Clancy, C. "Supplemental Insurance and Mortality in Elderly Americans." *Archives of Family Medicine,* 9 (2000): 251–7.

38. Blumenthal, David, "Controlling Health Care Expenditures." *NEJM,* 344 (10) (2001): 766–9.

39. Evans, R. G., "Authors Going for the Gold: the re-distributive agenda behind market-based healthcare reform." *Journal of Health Politics: Policy Law,* 2 (April 22, 1997): 475–96.

40. General Accounting Office, "Canadian Health Insurance Lessons for the United States." GAO/HRD (June 1991): 90–91.

41. <www.mms.org/physicians/resource/lewin.html> and <www.healthcareforall.com/lewincov.htm>.

42. Shiels, J; Haught, R. for The Lewin Group, Inc. "Analysis of the Costs and Impact of Universal Health Care Coverage Under a Single Payer Model for the State of Vermont." <http://www.dsw.state.vt.us/districts/ovha/AnalysisoftheCosts.pdf>. (8/28/01).

43. Himmelstein, David; Woolhandler, Steffie; Hellander, Ida. *Bleeding the Patient: The Consequences of Corporate Healthcare.* Common Courage Press, Monroe Maine. (2001): 83.

44. Mercer-Higgins, Foster, "National Survey of Employer-Sponsored Health Plans." *AMNews,* (January 22, 2001): 24.

45. Sager, Alan. "The Seven Myths Impeding Prescription Drug Reform in the United States." <http://dcc2.bumc.bu.edu/hs/ushealthreform.htm>. (8/15/01), and personal communication with Dr. Alan Sager.

46. OECD, Health Data 2000.

47. Ibid.

48. SAUS, 162 and 728 (2000).

49. OECD, Health Data 2000.

CHAPTER 8

1. OECD, Health Data 2000.

2. The weighted average was calculated by multiplying a nation's population size by the percentage of GDP spent on healthcare, summing these totals and then dividing by the total population of the nine comparison nations.

Weighted Average of the comparison nations as a percent of GDP spent on health care in 1998.

	Percent GDP expended on healthcare	Population (millions)	product	
Australia	8.5	18.7	158.95	
Canada	9.5	30.2	286.9	
France	9.6	58.9	565.44	
Germany	10.6	82	869.2	
Italy	8.4	56.9	477.96	
Japan	7.6	126.5	961.4	
Netherlands	8.6	15.7	135.02	
Spain	7.1	39.4	279.74	
United Kingdom	6.7	59.2	396.64	
		487.5	4131.25	8.47%

3. Calculated at 2.6 persons per household per Bureau of Census data Statistical Abstract of the United States (SAUS), 2000 table 62.

4. Berk, M; Monheit, A. "The Concentration of Health Care Expenditures, Revisited." *Health Affairs*, 20(2) (2001): 9–18.

5. Health Care Finance Administration, Health Care Financing Review Winter 1999 as in SAUS 2000, tables 151 and 152.

6. OECD, Health Data 2000.

7. OECD, Health Data 2000 and <http://dcc2.bumc.bu.edu/hs/ushealthreform.htm>. The revenues of prescription pharmaceuticals are somewhat difficult to perceive. The OECD reports total revenue to the industry of $82 billion from shipments in the US for 1998 while another reference reports $91 billion. HCFA reports expenditures of $121.9 billion for 1998, but includes drugs plus "other medical non-durables" at retail. This is in SAUS 2000 table 152. The Census Bureau in Current Industrial Reports (SAUS 2000,Table 1248) shows shipments of $65.5 billion in 1998 of pharmaceutical preparations except biologicals.

8. *Consumer Reports*, (October, 1993): 673.

9. AARP <www.aarp.org/cgi-bin/myaarp/articledetail>.

10. Pharmaceutical Industry General and Administrative expense outside of research and marketing is higher than the norm for American industry probably due to the high salaries for well qualified people; the need for well qualified consultant assistance, extensive government relations activity in a professional sense, and substantial travel and convention and meeting expenses.

11. OECD, Health data 2000.

12. The estimate of higher pharmaceutical pricing in the U.S. is partially based on the report of the Canadian Patented Medicine Prices Review Board Eleventh Annual Report, Year ending Dec 31, 1988, Ottawa. The results from p. 21 of this reference are in figure four.

There are many anecdotal reports of the differences Americans pay in the U.S. vs. other nations. There are anomalies in the PMPRB data. Assuming sales of ethical drugs were $91 billion in 1998 and the after tax profits of the manufacturers were 18.7% of revenue as referenced, then pre tax profits assuming a federal tax of 17% plus state taxes of 6% of EBT this must have been about $21.9 billion. The gross profit assuming fully burdened manufacturing cost and given the report of a 35% selling general and administrative expense would have been $69.2 billion. The reported 22% selling and marketing expense would have been $20.2 billion and other SG&A $ 9.9 billion. Fully burdened production costs were $21.8 billion. Research according to the OECD was $17.2 billion.

The OECD reports gross capital formation of the US industry rising from $2.5 billion in 1990 to $5.6 billion in 1995 the latest year for the data.

Assuming this data represents the generality and accepting the high profits as a reward for the high risks then overcharging in America may be going on in the unregulated market, but the funds are being used to advance the industry and its value to the society. There is excessive marketing expense in the competition as indicated in the text. In the macro analysis of the industry it does not seem possible that the overcharging could be more than 20% or $16.4 billion and is probably less. These funds are used both as marketing and research. To attribute $24.7 billion related to the industry as part of the excess expense of Americans is probably overstating. As is recommended in the final proposal these profit levels would be sustained under a single payer system assuming a reduction in marketing expenses. See the reference on the pharmaceutical industry in Chapter 10.

13. Health Care Financing Administration, (HCFA) *Health Care Financing Review*, (winter 1999) SAUS 2000, Table 152 but use rather the ratio of income from the AMA survey to determine practice expenses.

14. American Medical Association, Survey of Physicians. There is an anomaly between the Census of Business data and the AMA as to physicians' income. In a visit with Sara Thans of the AMA who is in charge of the survey, Olin Frederick was advised not to use a projection of income based on the AMA data due to uncertainties in the sample. Income data was also available from OECD. Since nearly two-thirds of U.S. physicians are specialists, it was determined that the ratio of income to practice expense would be representative of the specialists in the US. This has been used for all doctors.

15. Physicians income in other nations as reported by the OECD for the latest years shown follows in national currency units and U.S. dollars at the exchange rate: Op. cit OECD.

Nation	Year	Avg. Income		Avg. in U.S. $
USA	1996	USD	199,000	199,000
Australia	1997	AUD	72,727	56,877
Canada	1992	CAD	129,000	106,611
France	1997	FRF	404,285	69,346
Germany	1993	DEM	216,729	130,559
Japan	1997	JPY	10,182,684	77,795
United Kingdom	1999	GPB	28,265	45,588
Average	The latest year of the Comparison nations reporting:			81,129
Others				
Belgium	1993	BEF	1,719,544	49,812
Sweden	1995	SEK	398,364	55,877
Switzerland	1998	CHF	165,000	113,793

There are some caveats to this data. The income of Japanese physicians is understated since they also gain income from the sale of prescriptions drugs to their patients. The income of practicing physicians in U.K. is probably understated since their salaries are averaged with all physicians, even those in all stages of training. In 1991 the figure for the U.K. was USD 53,341. We believe the incomes in France, Belgium and Sweden are also understated possibly for the same reason. With this scattered data, and considering the caveats it is reasonable to conclude that American Physicians earn about twice the incomes of those in the comparison nations.

16. HCFA/SAUS, table 151.

17. Health Insurance Association of America, Washington DC: Health Insurance Data Annual. SAUS 2000, table 848.

18. Calculated from the HCFA data in SAUS 2000 table 152. This is the difference from the for-profit underwriting margin plus the known HCFA administrative expenses for Medicare at 2.2% of Medicare or $4.4 billion plus half that amount for all other tax supported programs.

19. Various amounts are given in various publications for the administration of Medicare. The amount of 2.2% was used recognizing a portion of the administrative costs are passed forward to insurance companies and providers to handle the payments and follow the regulations.

20. OECD, Health Data 2000.

21. OECD, Health Data 2000.

22. Woolhandler, Steffie MD and Himmelstein, David, MD, "The Deteriorating Administrative Efficiency of the U.S. Health Care System." *New England Journal of Medicine*, 324 (5) (1991): 1253–1258.

23. National Center for Health Statistics.

24. OECD, Health Data 2000.

25. Commonwealth Fund Survey, (1998). <http://www.cmwf.org/index.asp>.

26. OECD, Health Data 2000.

27. OECD, Health Data 2000.

28. *NEJM*, 324 (1991): 89–93.

29. OECD, Health Data 2000.

30. <www.phrma.org>. (3/15/01).

31. OECD, Health Data 2000.

32. OECD, Health Data 2000.

33. National Center for Health Statistics.

34. Dept Health and Human Services' Office of Inspector General. House Budget Committee Health Care Task Force: Medicare Program—Reducing Improper Payments and Fraud.

35. *Consumer Reports*, (September 2000).

36. Berk, M., "The Concentration of Health Expenditures: An Update." *Health Affairs*, (April 11, 1992): 145–149.

37. Health Care Financial Review, "Statistic Supply." (1997).

38. CDC. "Effectiveness in Disease and Injury Prevention Estimated National Spending on Prevention—United States, 1988." *MMWR*, 41 (29) (1992): 529–31.

39. <www.statehealthfacts.kff.org>. (6/1/01).

40. CDC. *Epidemiology and Prevention of Vaccine Preventable Diseases*, 6th Edition, 2nd printing. (January, 2001).

41. Ayanian, John Z. MD, MPP. Weissman, Joel S. PhD. Schneider, Eric C. MD, MSc. Ginsburg, Jack A. MPE. Zaslavsky, Alan M. PhD "Unmet Health Needs of Uninsured Adults in the United States." *JAMA*, 284 (16) (October 25, 2000): 2061–9.

42. National Center for Health Statistics.

43. Brownlee, Shannon, *Washington Post*, (March 6, 2001): HE10.

44. Lu, Michael C. MD, MPH. Lin, Yvonne G. MS. Prietto, Noelani M. MD. Garite, Thomas J. MD "Elimination of public funding of prenatal care for undocumented immigrants in California: A cost/benefit analysis." *Am Jr Ob Gyn*, 182 (2000): 233–9.

45. OECD, Health Data 2000.

46. Lewandowski K, Metz J, Detschmann H., et. al., "Incidence, severity, and mortality of acute respiratory failure in Berlin, Germany." *American Journal Respiratory Critical Care Medicine*, 151 (1995): 1121–1125.

47. Luhr O, Antonsen K, Karsson M. et. al. "Incidence and mortality after acute respiratory failure and acute respiratory distress syndrome in Sweden, Denmark, and Iceland." *American Journal Respir. Crit. Care Medicine*, 159 (1999): 1849–1861.

48. Behrendt, Carolyn E., PhD. *American College of Chest Physicians*, 118(4) (October 2000): 1100–1105.

49. Lewandowski K, Metz J, Detschmann H., et. al., "Incidence, severity, and mortality of acute respiratory failure in Berlin, Germany." *American Journal Respiratory Critical Care Medicine*, 151 (1995): 1121–1125.

50. Luhr O, Antonsen K, Karsson M. et. al. "Incidence and mortality after acute respiratory failure and acute respiratory distress syndrome in Sweden, Denmark, and Iceland." *American Journal Respir. Crit. Care Medicine*, 159 (1999): 1849–1861.

51. *Archives of Pediatric and Adolescent Medicine,* 154 (2000): 287–93.

52. OECD, Health Data 2000.

53. OECD, Health Data 2000.

545.National Institutes of Health (NIH), Global Initiative for COPD. <www.nhlbi.nih.gov/nhlbi/sciin//other/cht-book/htm>.

55. The Bulletin of the World Health Organization, (April 2000).

56. Goldman, Larry; Nielsen, Nancy; Champion, Hunter. "Awareness, Diagnosis, and Treatment of Depression." *Jr Gen Int Med.,* 14 (9) (1999): 569–80.

57. "US Emergency Dept. Costs: No Emergency." *Am Jr Pub Health,* (1996).

58. Salganik, William M., *The Baltimore Sun,* (January 31, 2001).

59. Nish, John; Chaturvedi, Jarrett; Shipley, Martin; Fuller, John. "Socioeconomic gradient in morbidity and mortality in people with diabetes: cohort study findings from the Whitehall study and the WHO multinational study of vascular disease in diabetes." *British Medical Journal,* 316 (7125) (January 1998): 100–105.

60. CDC, National Center for Chronic Disease Prevention and Health Promotion. <www.cdc.gov/cancer/index.htm>.

61. Wagner, Edward H. MD, MPH. Sandhu, Nirmala MPH. Newton, Katherine M. PhD. McCulloch, David K. MD. Ramsey, Scott D. MD, PhD. Grothaus, Louis C. MS. "Effect of Improved Glycemic Control on Health Care Costs and Utilization." JAMA, 285 (2) (January 10, 2001): 182–9.

62. Health for All of Western New York, Inc., "Health Risk Assessment Survey." (1999).

63. Congressional Budget Office, 2000.

64. Pear, Robert, *The New York Times,* "Budget Office's Estimates for Drug Spending Growth." (February 24, 2001).

65. OECD, Health Data 2000.

66. OECD, Health Data 2000.

67. Ayanian, John Z. MD, MPP. Weissman, Joel S. PhD. Schneider, Eric C. MD, MSc. Ginsburg, Jack A. MPE. Zaslavsky, Alan M. PhD "Unmet Health Needs of Uninsured Adults in the United States." JAMA, 284 (16) (October 25, 2000): 2061–9.

68. Ritz, Eberhard; Orth, Stephan." Primary Care: Nephropathy in Patients with Type 2 Diabetes Mellitus." *NEJM,* 341 (October 7, 1999): 1127–33.

69. U.S. Renal Data System.

70. *Am J Kid Dis,* 30 (2 Supplement 1) (1997): S40–53.

71. OECD, Health Data 2000.

72. The Global Lower Extremity Amputation Study Group Epidemiology of lower extremity amputation in centers in Europe, North America and East Asia. *British Journal of Surgery,* 87 (3) (March 2000): 328–337.

73. The Centers For Disease Control And Prevention. (CDC) "Total Tooth Loss Among Persons Aged >or= to 65 Years—Selected States, 1995–1997." JAMA, 281 (14) (April 14, 1999): 1264–1266.

74. CDC <www.cdc.gov/mmwr/preview/mmwrhtml/00056796.htm>. Ten Great Public Health Achievements—United States, 1900–1999." MMWR, 48 (1999): 241–243.

75. CDC. "Total Tooth Loss Among Persons Aged >or= to 65 Years—Selected States, 1995–1997." JAMA, 281 (14) (April 14, 1999): 1264–1266.

76. Nrderyd, Ola "Risk of severe periodontal disease in a Swedish adult population: A longitudinal study." *Journal of Clinical Peridontology,* 26 (9) (September 1999): 608–615.

77. Tiejian Wu, MD, PhD; Maurizio Trevisan, MD, MS; Robert J. Genco, DDS, PhD; Joan P. Dorn, PhD; Karen L. Falkner, PhD; Christopher T. Sempos, PhD "Periodontal Disease and Risk of Cerebrovascular Disease The First National Health and Nutrition Examination Survey and Its Follow-up Study." *Arch Internal Medicine,* 160 (2000): 2749–2755.

78. Oparil, Suzanne "Cardiovascular Health at the Crossroads: Outlook for the 21st Century: Presented at the 67th Scientific Sessions of the American Heart Association November 4, 1994 Dallas, Texas." *Circulation*, 91(4) (February 15, 1995): 1304–10.

79. Broderick J, Brott T, Kothari R, et al. "The Greater Cincinnati/ Northern Kentucky Stroke Study; preliminary first-ever and total incidence rates among blacks." *Stroke*, 29 (1998): 415–21.

80. *Stroke Connection Magazine*, (May/June 2000): 9.

81. *Stroke Connection Magazine*, (May/June 2000): 9.

82. *American Journal of Cardiology*, 83 (1999): 3A–4A.

83. Wilhelmsen, L; Rosengren, A; Eriksson, H; Lappas, G. "Heart failure in the general population of men—morbidity, risk factors and prognosis." *J Int Med*, 249 (3) (2001): 253–61.

84. Oparil, Suzanne "Cardiovascular Health at the Crossroads: Outlook for the 21st Century: Presented at the 67th Scientific Sessions of the American Heart Association November 4, 1994 Dallas, Texas." *Circulation*, 91 (4) (February 15, 1995): 1304–10.

85. OECD, Health Data 2000.

86. *Medical Care*, 37 (1999): 994–1012.

87. Cooper, Richard MD.; Cutler, Jeffrey MD. et.al. "Trends and Disparities in Coronary Heart Disease, Stroke, and Other Cardiovascular Diseases in the United States: Findings of the National Conference on Cardiovascular Disease Prevention." *Circulation*, 102 (2000): 3137–47.

88. Sarti C, Rastenytre D et al. "International Trends in Mortality from Stroke 1968–1994." *Stroke*, 31 (2000): 1588–1601.

89. Stephenson, Joan PhD. "UN Conference Endorses Battle Plan for HIV/AIDS." JAMA, 286 (4) (2001): 405–6.

90. OECD, Health Data 2000.

91. <www.statehealthfacts.kff.org>. (6/1/01).

92. OECD, Health Data 2000.

93. *Substance Abuse: The Nation's Number One Health Problems*, Schnieder Inst. For Health Policy, Branden University, (February 2001).

94. Banta, H. David MD, MPH. "Global Issues on the Agenda at the World Health Assembly: Discussion of HIV/AIDS, Leprosy, Access to Drugs." JAMA, 286 (1) (2001): 29.

95. Stephenson, Joan PhD. "UN Conference Endorses Battle Plan for HIV/AIDS." JAMA, 286 (4) (2001): 405–6.

96. Folkers, Gregory K. MS, MPH. Fauci, Anthony S. MD. "The AIDS Research Model: Implications for Other Infectious Diseases of Global Health Importance." JAMA, 286 (4) (2001): 458–61.

97. Banta, H. David MD, MPH. "Global Issues on the Agenda at the World Health Assembly: Discussion of HIV/AIDS, Leprosy, Access to Drugs." JAMA, 286 (1) (2001): 29.

98. Report from the American Diabetes Association." Economic Consequences of Diabetes Mellitus in the U.S. in 1997." *Diabetes Care*, 21 (2) (1998): 296–309.

99. OECD, Health Data 2000.

100. Ibid.

101. OECD, Health Data 2000.

102. *Consumer Reports*, (September 2000).

103. Ayanian, John Z. MD, MPP. Weissman, Joel S. PhD. Schneider, Eric C. MD, MSc. Ginsburg, Jack A. MPE. Zaslavsky, Alan M. PhD "Unmet Health Needs of Uninsured Adults in the United States." JAMA, 284 (16) (October 25, 2000): 2061–9.

104. Ibid.

CHAPTER 9

1. *Newsweek*, (February 12, 2001): 38–43.
2. *The Post-Journal*, "Pataki Promises Reforms of New York Drug Laws." (January 4, 2001).
3. CDC. "Ten Great Public Health Achievements—United States, 1900–1999." *MMWR*, 48 (12) (1999): 1.
4. McGinnis, J. Michael. Foege, William H. "Actual Causes of Death in the United States." *JAMA*, 270 (18) (November 10, 1993): 2207–2212.
5. NCC *Disease Prevention*.
6. *Substance Abuse: The Nation's Number One Health Problems*, Schnieder Inst. For Health Policy, Branden University, (February 2001).
7. *The Post-Journal*, "Pataki Promises Reforms of New York Drug Laws." (January 4, 2001).
8. Meenan, Dr. Robert, *Boston Globe*, (November 3, 2000).
9. *The Post-Journal*, AP Newswire, (June 28,2001).
10. Mauer, M., "Young Black Americans and the Criminal Justice System: Five Years Later." Wash DC *The Sentencing Project*. 9070 (1995).
11. Vastag, Brian. "Federal Plan Asks for Increased Drug Treatment." *JAMA*, 284(24) (2000): 3114.
12. Erica Goode, *The New York Times*, "9 Million Gaining Upgraded Benefit for Mental Care." (January 1, 2001).
13. Meenan, Dr. Robert, *Boston Globe*, (November 3, 2000).
14. The Bulletin of the World Health Organization, (April 2000).
15. U.S. Bureau of the Census, Statistical Abstract of the United States (1996).
16. *The Nursing Facility Sourcebook*, "1998 Executive Summary."
17. American Healthcare Association.
18. The Nursing Facility Sourcebook, "1998 Executive Summary."
19. HCFA's Online Survey, Certification and Reporting Date, (March 1997).
20. Harrington, Charlene; Woolhandler, Steffie; Mullan, Joseph; Carrillo, Helen; Himmelstein, David. "Quality of Care Lower in For-Profit, Investor-Owned Nursing Homes." *Am Jr Public Health*, 91 (9) (2001): 1–5.
21. Van Nostrand, Joan F., Clark, Robert F. and Inge Romoren, Tor, "Nursing Home Care in Five Nations." *Journal of the International Federation on Ageing*; Aging International: Long-Term Care Challenges in an Aging World, XX (2) (June 1993): 1–5.
22. MSSNY *News of New York*, (December 2000): 6.
23. AMPAC report, Center for Responsive Politics, *AMNews*, (January 22, 2001): 9.
24. Landers, Steven; Sehgal, Ashwini. "How Do Physicians Lobby Their Members of Congress?" *Arch Intern Med*, 160 (November 27, 2000): 3248–3251.
25. Hamburger/McGinley, *The Wall Street Journal*, (November 9, 2000).
26. <http://commoncause.org/publications/june01/phrma/061201.pdf>.
27. *Worst Pills/Best Pills*, 7 (6) (2001): 47.
28. Bayoy, Jennifer, *Boston Globe*, (July 24,001).
29. Peter Honig, MD., Personal Communication. (July 7, 2001).
30. AMPAC report, Center for Responsive Politics. *AMNews*, (January 22,2001): 9.
31. Levy, Clifford, *The New York Times*, (February 5, 2001).
32. Taylor, S., "Tobacco Lawyers and the Case for Cover-up Reform." *National Journal Group*, (2001).
33. Fox, Daniel; Fronstin, Paul. "Public Spending for Health Care Approaching 60%." *Health Affairs*, 19 (2) (2000): 271–3.

34. <www.statehealthfacts.kff.org>. (6/1/01).

35. Parment, William L. Assemblyman and the NYS Comptroller's Office, Personal Communication, (January 3, 2001).

36. Teresi, Samuel, Mayor Jamestown, NY, Personal Communication.

37. <www.statehealthfacts.kff.org>. (6/1/01).

38. <www.statehealthfacts,kff.org>. (6/1/01).

CHAPTER 10

1. Campion, Edward W. "A Symptom of Discontent." *NEJM*, 344 (3) (2001): 223–5.

2. OECH Health Data 2000.

3. Pastoral Letter on Healthcare, Joseph Cardinel Bernardin (October 1995).

4. NBC News/*The Wall Street Journal*, (October, 23–5, 1999). <www.pollingreport.com/health>.

5. Michaud, C; Murray, C.: Bloom, B "Burden of Disease—Implications for Future Research." *JAMA*, 285 (5) (2/7/01): 535–9.

6. Long S.H., "Universal Health Insurance and Uninsured People: Effects on Use and Cost: Report to Congress." Washington, D.C., Office of Tech. Assessment and Congressional Research Survey, Library of Congress, (August 5, 1994); Figure 1:4.

7. The definition of "healthcare expenses" is not clear in the reference. The total used is for services "received" by patients as opposed to total expenditure. This leaves out the elements of health care not directly related to patient care, specifically public health, research, construction and the insurance administration. It also excludes dentistry. See SAUS 2000, tables 151/2.

8. Ayanian, John Z. MD, MPP. Weissman, Joel S. PhD. Schneider, Eric C. MD, MSc. Ginsburg, Jack A. MPE. Zaslavsky, Alan M. PhD "Unmet Health Needs of Uninsured Adults in the United States." *JAMA*, 284 (16) (October 25, 2000): 2061–9.

9. A macro analysis of the pharmaceutical industry in the U.S. was used to estimate that profit levels could be maintained with a substantial volume increase. The industry fears a single payer, which will have the ultimate bargaining power. However, policy should be included in enabling legislation that requires the single payer to guarantee high profits to the industry in return for the risks it takes. This policy should also insist on reduced marketing expenses with a means of providing more effective communication with doctors concerning new drugs or therapies. Universal care will reduce the need for samples and accord to them their intended use, for patient tolerance. The macro analysis is based on surveys and OECD data. In 1998 sales of pharmaceuticals in the U.S. were $ 91 billion. The profit of the industry was 18.7% of revenue after taxes. The federal tax was 17% of revenue. Marketing was 22% of revenue and research was $17.2 billion. Total Selling, General and Administrative (SG&A) expense including marketing but not including research was 35% of revenue. This allows the following analysis of a macro income statement, which does not include inventory adjustments:

TOTAL	1998 actual	1998 with NHP
Net Revenue	$ 91.0	$ 113.75
Variable production cost:	13.1	16.4
Fixed production cost:	8.7	8.7
Fully burdened production cost:	21.8	25.1
Gross profit:	69.2	88.7
SG&A		
Marketing:	20.2	11.4
Other	9.9	11.0
Reduced marketing		10.9
Research	17.2	17.2
Earnings before interest and taxes:	21.9	38.2
Allowance for taxes:	5.0	8.8
Net profit after tax:	16.9	29.4

It is important to emphasize that this analysis pictures the very best of the companies with the lesser performers. This is a complex industry dealing in a complex scientific discipline. It has been productive beyond the imagination of most observers. Not much should be changed. The marketing excesses are the main issue. Testing against the standard therapies for cost or effectiveness improvement is a question for debate.

10. World Health Organization Report 2000. <www.who.int>.

11. This statement assumes that hospitals billed the $60 billion but couldn't collect. Through their budgeting processes hospitals and doctors can assume much of their billings will not be paid. They then raise their charges to cover their costs. In the case of the $60 billion, hospitals budgeted $382 billion and overcharged to get it. Had they not, their revenues would have been $ 322 billion. The overcharge was 18.6% or $60 billion but that is probably not the total shortfall. Estimates can be as high as one-third or $127 billion.

12. The matrix shows the effect of the assumptions and the calculations of economic effect from Chapter 8.

Total expenditure is reduced by the amount of investment in facilities. It is assumed that the amortization for previous investment is in the current accounts and the new investment is paid by financing. This item really does not belong in the expenditures, but government accountants frequently place it there. Even if the investment were paid from current cash flow, it would still have to be capitalized. The investment is also deducted from the payments. This is the suspected correction the OECD makes in determining total expenditure as noted in Chapter 8. The OECD gives the U.S. total health expenditure as $1,129 billion as opposed to the HCFA 1,149.1 billion in 1998.

New Rights are those as calculated under the estimated start-up costs.

Retraining relates to the displacement of employees of doctors offices, hospitals and insurance companies. In 1999 according to the Bureau of Labor Statistics there were 9,973,000 employees in health services including 1,865,000 in doctor's offices; 3,970,000 in hospitals; 1,755,000 in nursing homes and personal care facilities; and 655,000 in home care.(SAUS 2000, table 684) There were 4,090,000 professionals including 720,000 doctors, 173,000 dentists, 2,128,000 registered nurses and 216,000 pharmacists. Total employment in insurance was 1,635,000 in the carriers and 767,000 in agencies and broker firms and related services. The displacement will be in doctors offices and hospitals in which personnel will shift from administration to care giving assuming 90% of the persons with new rights for care take advantage of them. A large displacement is also expected in health insurance. The number of persons working in health insurance in both for-profit and not-for-profit organizations is not clear. The estimate is that 1,500,000 will be shifted to care giving or related pursuits. Their salaries are continued. The cost shown is for their educational expenses.

Tuition carries out the recommendation of paying for the education of students who accept places in medical and dental schools.

Nurses increase carries out the recommendation to increase nurses' salaries. In the base year of 1998, the average nurse salary was estimated at $37,000 based on various data sources.

NHP SAVINGS are those calculated in Chapter 8 as excess expenses. The reduction of the cost of sick people who should not be sick commences at 10% the first year and the at 15% of the original amount in the successive years. It is assumed that some are cured; some die; and increasingly fewer "underclass" patients become ill. The savings in pharmaceutical marketing excesses is separate. This and the other savings are held constant at the 1998 amount.

PAYMENTS are the out-of-pocket and tax supported payments into the system.

The out-of-pocket amount is half the real amount for 1998 and increases at 1.86%.

The Present Tax Support includes every category except Medicare, which is shown separately. These are from HCFA (SAUS 2000 tables 151/2) The items marked * are the estimated shares.

The totals are given in the source.

Federal:

Federal Share of Medicaid	$74.8 billion*
Public Health, CDC and NIH	17.0*
Military hospitals	13.6
Maternal and child programs	2.6
Veterans Administration	17.1
Research	18.3
Medical Vocational Rehabilitation	.8
Federal Total	$144.2

State and Local:

Share of Medicaid and other aid:	$100.7 billion
Workmen's compensation	17.0
State and local hospitals	11.8
Temporary disability	.1
Public health	19.6*
Misc.	8.7
State and local total	$157.9

In addition to these items all governments, including the federal, pay for their employees private health insurance. The total expended by all governments for this purpose was $67.3 billion or about $3273 per employee. Since this is tax supported, the tax total excluding Medicare is $369.4 billion.

The other private payments are university or philanthropic research.

The balance of the matrix assumes the substitution of the NHP tax for private payments. This nets most of the immediate savings by eliminating the present multi-payer insurance system thus reducing costs in the 1998 model by $90 billion. Net private payments for insurance plus one half the out-of-pocket and other programs totaled $513.6 billion in 1998. The NHP tax calculates to $ 448.9 billion or $ 64.7 billion less than what individuals actually paid.

13. Commonwealth Fund Survey, (1998): <www.cmwf.org/index.asp>.

14. <www.statehealthfacts.kff.org>. (6/1/01).

15. *The Post-Journal*, (July 17, 2001): 1.

INDEX OF ECONOMIC AND STATISTICAL DATA